The Yin & Yang Lifestyle Guide

Michael Hetherington
(L.Ac & Yoga Teacher)

First Published 2014
Mind Heart Publishing

www.mindheartpublishing.com

Australia

Disclaimer

All material in this book is provided for your information only and may not be construed as medical advice or instruction. No action or inaction should be taken based solely on the contents of this information; instead, readers should consult appropriate health professionals on any matter relating to their health and well-being.

The information and opinions expressed here are believed to be accurate, based on the best judgment available to the authors, and readers who fail to consult with appropriate health authorities assume the risk of any injuries. The publisher is not responsible for errors or omissions.

About the Author

Michael Hetherington is a qualified acupuncturist, lecturer in Oriental medicine and yoga teacher based in Brisbane, Australia. He has a keen interest in mind-body medicine, energetic anatomy, nutrition and herbs, yoga nidra and Buddhist-style meditation. Inspired by the teachings of many, he has learned that a light-hearted, joyful approach to life serves best.

www.michaelhetherington.com.au

Other Titles by Author:

The Complete Book of Oriental Yoga

Meditation Made Simple

How to Do Restorative Yoga

Chakra Balancing Made Simple and Easy

The Little Book of Yin

How to Learn Acupuncture

Table of Contents

Introduction

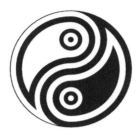

"Those who flow as life flows know they need no other force."
~ Lao Tzu

Many of us have come across the theory of yin and yang at some point in our lives, and we may be familiar with how it is used to explain various opposing forces and extremes in our natural world. They are often expressed in contrasts, such as sun and moon, light and dark, male and female. However, the theory of yin and yang can be explored to much greater depths and explored in a way that can be applied more pragmatically to our daily lives in a way that enhances and encourages overall balance, healing, stability, and, ultimately, serenity of mind.

Within the pages of this book, we will go deeper into the theory of yin and yang and how this theory is strongly associated to our health, our well-being, and our spiritual development. There is also a quiz in the *Yin and Yang Quiz* chapter that you can complete to help you have a better understanding as to whether you may have more yin or yang characteristic in your life at this current time and what you can do to bring things back to a balanced state.

The primary purpose of this book is to develop a deeper understanding of the forces of yin and yang and to give practical suggestions as to how to go about working with the forces of yin and yang rather than against them. The term or theory of "balance" will also be discussed, as it is not often clear as to what balance is and how being in balance feels.

Learning to flow with yin and yang sets can be one of the greatest adventures of one's life, for when one if "synced up" to these cosmic forces, life takes on a smoother and more fluid unfolding in a way that is nurturing, supportive, and naturally produces a deeper sense of appreciation.

What is Yin and Yang?

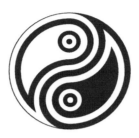

"The creation of a thousand forests is in one acorn."
~ Ralph Emerson

Yin and Yang is a symbol and metaphor for the two most fundamental forces found in Nature. It is hailed as one of the greatest concepts and philosophical ideas put forward by ancient Chinese philosophers and naturalists.

The earliest Chinese characters representing yin and yang were found as inscriptions on "oracle bones", the skeletal remains of animals, which are believed to have been used as part of Chinese divination practices from at least 1300BC. The inscription of yin and yang on these bones literally translated in reference to the movements of the sun. Yang was translated as the sunny side of the mountain, and yin was the shady side of the mountain. Therefore, these early signs of yin and yang theory were very much in relation to sun based movements and cycles. Interestingly, no one has ever claimed to be the originator and founder of the yin and yang symbol we are now familiar with.

Around the time of the Spring and Autumn period (770-481BC), and the Warring States period (403-221BC) in China, there existed a school of scholarly thought, which came to be called the yinyang school. The yinyang school focused on the study and observation of how yin and yang expressed itself in nature as well how yin and yang expressed itself in man. These scholars observed and recorded the cycles found in the natural world and in modern day terms, this field of scholarly pursuit would be considered to be some kind of natural science. Along with the yinyang school were 5 other schools of scholarly thought at the time, Confucian, Mohist, Legalist, Fatalist, and Daoist. It was during these periods that the yinyang school is believed to have thrived as well as expanded into other related fields of study. They developed the 5 element theory, which is still used in Traditional Chinese medicine today and they also worked upon calendar keeping, the study of numbers, astronomy, and divination. It is believed that many of the great books and writings that were produced during the peak of the yinyang school have not survived. After these golden periods in Chinese philosophical history, many of the schools of scholarly thought either dissolved or merged into each other. It appears that the yinyang school merged into what we now call neo-Confucianism, which focuses more on moral and ethical philosophies governed primarily by reason.

From the original framework of yin and yang theory was born the I Ching, more commonly known as "the book of changes". The I Ching is considered one of the oldest Chinese divination type systems, which is believed to have been formulated sometime before 1000BC. The I Ching takes the simplified yin and yang theory and expands it into 64 hexagrams 6 layers deep, all displaying various combinations of yin and yang. The I Ching attempts to explain and explore all the possible varying cycles of nature, expressed as time or phases that the human being travels through. Time in this philosophical framework is never seen as linear, but rather, cyclic, much like the change of the seasons.

According to the I Ching, human beings travel through only 64 various expressions or phases of time, each phase their own strengths and weaknesses, according to the variations and influences of yin and yang forces. The I Ching was, and still is, used as a system of divination to help one identify what current time phase one is in and the I Ching serves as a kind of guide to assist us in our current decision making processes and daily affairs.

Another interesting observation coming out of the yinyang school was the belief and observation that the universe, according to this yin yang theory, is essentially morally aligned. Meaning that any acts, such as violence, greed, and so on, are to automatically against the universal flow of things and, therefore, only leads one away from being able to live a healthy, virtuous, and peaceful life.

The yin and yang approach, in relation to how to live a good and healthy life, is primarily focused on the practice of avoiding extremes of either yin or yang energies, for to do so only invites disaster. For example, the yin and yang theory is used in the field of human health and medicine, more specifically, Traditional Chinese Medicine. Yin and yang is applied in Chinese medicine as a way to help us *predict* certain outcomes in the cases of illness. Yin and yang can also serve as a warning so that if we detect any extreme, we can adjust our behaviors to avoid an illness or some kind of calamity. When we are able to see the yin and yang patterns expressing themselves in life, we can more consciously implement various strategies as a way to shift from any unhealthy yin or yang pattern as a means to help correct any potential of imbalance. When extremes are avoided, we tend to avoid unnecessary illness, drama, or disaster as life takes on a more fluid form of expression.

Natural laws are in place, whether or not we believe in them and whether or not we choose to accept them. Just like gravity implies its own forces upon us, we can accept this force and work with it or we can try to ignore it and go against it. Any sensible person knows that to attempt to go against the force of gravity is futile and would only drain us of our efforts until we were to succumb to the truth of to its influence and recognize it as physical reality. Where physics is an attempt to understand the physical laws of nature, yin and yang may be considered as a simplified way to understand the universal laws of nature of both the physical world and the subtler energetic world.

All of these natural laws exist without our choosing and so the sensible person is advised to study and learn about these forces from a young age so that when one comes of age, they can act in the world with wisdom and intelligence with full knowing as to the natural forces present. This is the primary purpose of schooling, is it not? We are taught about many things like science, mathematics, languages, cultures, and so on, in an attempt to equip us with the basic understandings as to how this world "ticks". When we have a good grounding and understanding in these ways, we are surely well equipped to work with them and, hopefully, flourish in this world. Unfortunately, I have observed that there are many natural universal laws that we tend not to be taught in our educational system, which would be a great benefit to help us, as human flourish later in life. One of the most obvious and alarming problems in our human societies is the issue of stress, mental illness, depression, and obesity. All of these manifestations tend to come out of the one natural occurring phenomenon of which we are taught little to nothing at school. What we are not taught about in school is the workings of our own minds. The study of the mind would include how to recognize stress patterns in our thinking, how food and exercise influence our psychology, how habits and environments influence our mind, and to be provided with a list of helpful and effective strategies that would help us manage and deal with emotions and mental processes. Were you ever taught or practiced any of these things in school? Do you think it would have been valuable to learn more about the workings of your own mind and some strategies to train and manage it more effectively?

Another important point regarding the forces of yin and yang is that these forces *are not personal.* They do not care what our opinions or beliefs are, for they yield the same power upon us regardless. Just like the movements of the sun adheres to certain laws of the physical domain, which are impersonal, so, too, does yin and yang operate in this way. Any natural law that is, is, regardless of our opinions or beliefs and therefore may be considered a universal truth and, therefore, is applicable to all humans regardless of race, religion, and cultural background.

Yang is commonly expressed as extreme heat, energy, expansion, sun, male energy, and so forth. Yin is commonly expresses at cold, passive, creative, moon, female energy, and so forth. The ancient Taoists discovered that all things, both animate and inanimate objects, can be broken down into primarily yin or yang characteristics. This process of breaking things down into two primary forces provided a context where the theory and notion of balance could be better understood. It also provided a way that could help humans navigate through the cosmic forces of the universe in a way that was aligned and supportive of its evolution.

The fundamental principle found in the theory of yin and yang is that even though all things can be categorized down to its basic yin or yang nature, it cannot explain things in absolute terms. To be in absolute terms would indicate that one thing was 100% yang and 0% yin or 100% yin and 0% yang, which, in its very definition, is not possible within yin and yang theory. For if something was 100% yang, yin would not exist or there would be no reason for it to exist. Thus, this presents us with a unique perspective into the world as all things depend on another for their very own existence. It also brings us toward a paradoxical principle that indicates that "it is, and it isn't". This means that it can be it and it can also not be it at the same time because nothing is completely 100% separate from its opposite. For there to be 'good', there also needs to be 'bad', because without the 'bad', it is not possible to know good and therefore, they both exist simultaneously. For life, there also needs to be death. For me to be me, I need you to be you because if you were to change in any way, it would also change me because we share both the yin and yang and are, in a very abstract way, very dependent on each other. Therefore, all variations and expressions of this world can only exist when there are variations of things that are not that. As an example, if we were all to share the same ideas and attitudes, the world would be very bland and boring place with no variation. Therefore, we need variation, we need both the 'good and the bad', we need death to experience life and thus, we come to the crux of this philosophy when we say: there is nothing fundamentally "wrong" in this universe and in the human experience. It is all interdependent, based on variations of various factors that makes up who you are and who I am. We are simply expressions of this universal law.

This understanding breaks us open and provides us with a deeper truth into the nature of yin and yang; that is, that the absolute is not able to be expressed, quantified, explained, or exemplified because the idea of yin and yang is as far as the human mind can go, as far as logical reasoning and the use of communication is concerned. This becomes more obvious when we look at language. For example, when we use a word, up, this implies automatically that there exists those things that are up, and those things that are not up, which means down, which is the dualistic nature of yin and yang. Without 'down', there would be no meaning the word 'up'. Therefore, our language is used via the principles of contrast and opposites to help us express our meaning. Once any word or symbol is used, it is automatically indicating that there is something that is not, and something that is, which highlights the fact that one word or symbol can never be absolute and all inclusive. On further investigation, it becomes obvious, according to this notion, that if the absolute can never be expressed through words or symbols, then it indicates that the absolute cannot be expressed or experienced through thought forms, either. Therefore, all thought forms, whether they be images or words, can also be viewed as incomplete and non-absolute, which, through this realization, although perhaps daunting at first, somewhat acts to help de-energize the contents of the mind. This is an important step and realization for any human to make, as it now gives us the opportunity to be able to step back from the importance placed on our mind's contents. What tends to drive the human mad is that he thinks his thoughts very, very important and, therefore, takes them very, very seriously. However, when we can see that thought forms are not absolute and incomplete, we are then invited to seek out what lays beyond the mind, and beyond all forms of categorization.

Before we can get to that stage, it seems that the path for many of us humans is that we must first travel through the objectification process of the mind, a kind of mental development, which we commonly refer to as education. This builds up the sophistication of the mind and intellect to a point that is may serve us well in worldly affairs. However, it also serves as a kind of trap, for many become transfixed in this mentally developed space, and what initially serves us through our process of evolution, can, after some time, strangle our growth to such an extent that evolution of the human understanding grinds to a halt and, in some cases, is unable to progress any further. Instead of becoming stuck in the limitations of the mental realm, it is beneficial to reach that point, which we will all reach at some point, where one has the opportunity to leap out and go beyond it. It takes courage to leap beyond the mind, yet any fears that exist as a means to resist you from doing so, dissolve into insignificance once the grand splendor of the space beyond the mind is revealed. If one does go beyond the mind, the mind and its functions are still available to us; so, in effect, we do not lose it, but we come to a space where it does not rule or govern us. This is a process of un-education, or re-education. A process commonly expressed in various schools of Buddhism, and Zen, in particular, where the practitioner actually learns to unlearn everything learned while remaining with a highly sophisticated intellectual capacity, and, in this way, becomes free from the limitations and trappings of the mind.

Until such time or opportunity, we are required to come back to develop our minds and study the alignment of the Yin and Yang as best as we can come to understand it. The study and alignment with yin and yang is a path that generates more virtue and peace in our daily affairs and allows natural wisdom to rise to the surface of our awareness. The following illustration expands upon the various qualities that can be found within yin and yang.

Yin 陰 陽 Yang

The theory of Yin and Yang is one of the greatest contributions of Chinese thought. The earliest reference to Yin and Yang is in the I Ching (Book of Changes) in approximately 700 BC. In this work, all phenomena are said to be reduced to Yin and Yang.

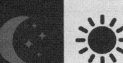

Yin	Yang
1. Darkness	1. Light
2. Moon	2. Sun
3. Passive	3. Active
4. Negative	4. Positive
5. Female	5. Male
6. Earth	6. Heaven
7. Matter	7. Energy
8. Blood	8. Qi
9. Shady Side	9. Sunny Side
10. Relaxation	10. Ambition

The Four Principles of Yin & Yang

1. Yin-Yang are opposites

They are either on the opposite ends of a cycle, like the seasons of the year, or, opposites on a continuum of energy or matter. This opposition is relative, and can only be spoken of in relationships.

2. Interdependent: Can not exist without each other

Nothing is totally Yin or totally Yang. Just as a state of total Yin is reached, Yang begins to grow. Yin contains seed of Yang and vise versa. They constantly transform into each other.

3. Mutual consumption of Yin and Yang

Relative levels of Yin Yang are continuously changing. Normally this is a harmonious change, but when Yin or Yang are out of balance they affect each other, and too much of one can eventually weaken and consume the other.

4. Inter-transformation of Yin and Yang

One can change into the other, but it is not a random event, happening only when the time is right.

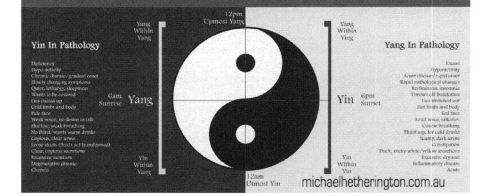

Yin In Pathology

Deficiency
Hypo-activity
Chronic disease/gradual onset
Slowly changing symptoms
Quiet, lethargy, sleepiness
Wants to be covered
Lies curled up
Cold limbs and body
Pale face
Weak voice, no desire to talk
Shallow, weak breathing
No thirst/wants warm drinks
Copious, clear urine
Loose stools (fluids not transformed)
Clear, copious secretions
Excessive moisture
Degenerative disease
Chronic

Yang In Pathology

Excess
Hyperactivity
Acute disease/rapid onset
Rapid pathological changes
Restlessness, insomnia
Throws off bedclothes
Lies stretched out
Hot limbs and body
Red face
Loud voice, talkative
Coarse breathing
Thirst esp. for cold drinks
Scanty, dark urine
Constipation
Thick, sticky white/yellow secretions
Excessive dryness
Inflammatory disease
Acute

michaelhetherington.com.au

The defining of objects into yin and yang depend completely on context. For example, you may say the sun is yang because of the color and heat radiating from it and the moon is yin because of its passive, quiet, and cold-like nature. However, if we are to change the context from comparing the sun to the moon, we may now compare the size and mass of the moon to the size and mass of Pluto. Which one is now more yin or yang? The moon would be more yang because it is much larger (over 5x), which then makes Pluto more yin then yang. So as you can see, yin and yang is completely dependent on context to decipher whether something is yin or yang. Generally speaking, however, on the human level, when comparing various environments for a human to live in, the food they consume, the movements they engage in, and the thought processes they have, there are common yin and yang elements that can established.

There are four primary principles of yin and yang and the relationship between the two. These four principles are the gateways into a more thorough understanding of yin and yang and, therefore, worth some further contemplation and discussion.

The four principles of Yin and Yang are:

1. Yin and Yang Oppose Each other

As a result of yin and yang's dynamic movement, this principle emphasizes that these forces are in a kind of interlocking, ongoing conflict. It often helps to visualize in your mind's eye, a giant electromagnetic field that stretches out as far as the imagination allows. Now imagine this electromagnetic field having waves and ripples flowing throughout it like the waves of the ocean. It is these waves and ripples of movement that generate phases and areas within this energetic web, great areas of conflict, or in other words, areas of great resistance. With any resistance, when left long enough, generates and stagnates a mass amount of potential energy until it reaches a tipping point, where the stagnant energy eventually overpowers the resistance force, which can generate a massive movement or release of energy. It is this quality of opposing yin and yang forces that brings to life dynamic periods of intensity, beauty, and sometimes destruction for the energy to be able to continue to move and adjust itself eventually back toward balance.

2. Yin and Yang mutually create and depend on each other

Yin and yang co-exist and are bound together in a co-dependent relationship. They only can exist as long as its partner, and opposing force, is also in existence. It is this interlocking, co-dependent relationship that give rise to their true definition and shows us that these forces cannot be separated. It is like man and woman, if you were to take away all the men on the planet, eventually all humans would cease to exist because they could no longer procreate. Therefore, man and woman are perfect expressions of the co-existing relationship found throughout the universe.

3. Yin and Yang change and grow in a cyclic and balanced manner

Yin and yang are always moving in a way to turn toward a more balanced state. It does this through the continuous dynamic movement of interaction and restriction. In Taoism, a philosophy grounded in the study and practice of yin and yang, views the universe to be self-governed. They feel that it is this yin and yang force that governs all of life, therefore, there is no God or entity outside of these forces to which is worthy of attention or that we can depend on to "fix our life", if, for some reason, it fell apart.

If one was to sit and observe these yin and yang forces expressing themselves throughout the natural world, we come to see yin and yang patterns start to emerge. The most obvious of these patterns is the changes of the weather and the four seasons. We would also see the patterns and cycles in the animal world as well as the human world, in relation to birth, the aging process, disease, and death. On deeper inspection, we may also be able to observe patterns in our behaviors and our thinking processes. Whatever we are viewing or observing, it will soon become obvious that it is indeed constantly changing and that if we watch long enough, a pattern would naturally emerge.

4. Yin and Yang transform into each other.

Hot will eventually become cold and cold will eventually become hot. There is simply no other way. Although it may take thousands or millions of years, such as an ice age here on Earth, it will still come to pass, where the sun will come to melt the ice. Nature has its own way of restoring balance, and according to universal time and space, nature is very, very patient. Another example can be seen right in front of us. We can see it unfolding in our breath. The inhale will eventually become exhale and vice versa. It is impossible to only inhale only, without the exhale. Therefore, these forces feed and support each other, giving opportunity for its opposite to be expressed and for life force to exist.

Yin, Yang and Change

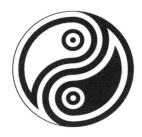

"The only way to make sense of change is to plunge into it, move with it, and join the dance." ~ Alan Watts

As mentioned earlier, one of the greatest teachings yin and yang can offer us is that everything is constantly changing. Yin and Yang are the perfect expression of this constantly changing phenomena, which is found throughout the external world as well as the internal world.

When we really come to understand and practice this law of change, we give up trying to hold onto things because we come to see that the more we hold on, the greater the anxiety of losing it. And so it is found that it is the simple, yet not easy, practice of letting go rather than holding on, which brings us peace. Holding on brings tension, letting go brings peace.

The first and most fundamental step in really embodying and syncing with this natural law is to first accept that all forms, which include sounds, images, thoughts, and emotions, change. Secondly, allow adaptation and flexibility for change to occur unhindered. And thirdly, syncing up with the natural flow of yin and yang "switches on" greater potentials of energy, insight, and understanding.

1. Accept that everything changes

Good times will change, bad times will change, relationships will change, and fortunes will change. Within the world of form, all has a limited time that it can blossom for. For it is in their impermanence that they can be enjoyed. Therefore, when boredom comes, be bored, when joy comes, be joyful, when sadness comes, be sad. A great deal of human anxiety and suffering kicks in when we are constantly trying to avoid, resist, or run away from what we are feeling and experiencing in the present moment. When we are running away, or unsatisfied with what is, right now, we are running away from life. So if we are continuously trying to run away from the present moment, we are running away from ourselves and away from truly living.

One approach to learning to accept and live with this constant change in our world is to continuously let everything go, all of the time. When we let go, we become more peaceful. The peace comes when we let go of trying to control or hold onto things, for to do so generates anxiety. Yet, when we let go, we come back into the present moment with what is and as we come back to the present moment, peacefulness arises, and where peacefulness is.

2. Allow for flexibility and adaption to change as it arises

Freedom comes from one's capacity to accept change and adapt to it as it arises in every moment. The tendency for humans is to seek out stability and avoid and resist any change that may threaten that sense of stability. This is setting oneself up for failure and disappointment because it is impossible to find true, lasting stability in this world, for it is always changing and moving because that is its nature. It is natural for the human to seek out stability and certainty but we look in the wrong places. We seek it in the outside world in the form of money, environment, relationships, and so on. The true stability and security we seek is inside, within our own heart. When we find true peace in our heart, we can be anywhere in the world, doing anything, and have the feeling of being unmoved. This is true stability. To seek it in the outside world is to give away our power, because we project our power outside. If we were to point that attention and power back into our heart, then we build and generate our own sanctuary. Eventually, this heart sanctuary becomes so strong and steady that we experience true stability. This is difficult for most of us because socially, we are largely directed and programmed to look outward for sources of stability. We look for jobs, places, and people to satisfy our desire for stability and although these things may provide comfort for some time, they will eventually dissolve and we are left hankering after the next thing. At some point, we will come to realize it was with us the entire time and is totally non-dependent on the world outside.

It is when we come to be established in this inner sanctuary that we are able too much more easily adapt and flex with the movements of the outside world without effort, strain, or resistance.

3. Adjust lifestyle to sync up with the natural cycles of yin and yang to give rise to greater power and insight.

It is always better to avoid extremes, as they tend to throw us around, quickly exhaust our energy, and disturb the mind. Learning to sync up with and honor the natural cycles and expressions of yin and yang teaches us humility in the face of cosmic law. When we learn to sync up and go with this natural force, we actually become more powerful because we tap into the universal flow of energy. Essentially, we ride the wave and this wave has an immense amount of power backing it. The more we learn to ride these cosmic waves, the more power and energy we have available. This boost of power amplifies our thoughts, intentions, and actions so that whatever we focus on, we enhance its capacity to actualize and manifest. Riding these cosmic waves also tends to bring some stability to the bodies functioning, and to the mind, which helps us move more easily into conducive states of meditation and contemplation.

The Notion of Balance

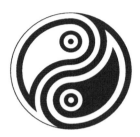

"Life is like riding a bicycle. To keep your balance, you must keep moving." ~ Albert Einstein

What is often alluded to in discussions of yin and yang theory is the notion of balance. Balance being a somewhat illusive ideal state in which yin and yang are harmonized, equalized, and equanimous. What is rarely discussed is, what does being balanced actually feel like, look like, and how do I know if I am balanced or not? What are the signs that present themselves when balance is present? And if one becomes balanced, does that translate as being enlightened?

Because of the nature of Yin and Yang, the state of balance between these forces is actually a very rare occurrence. So much so, that the very notion that one can stay in balance for any amount of time is not really possible, or at least for any great amount of time. Yin and yang is like the movements of the planets or the rising and falling of the tides. Every now and then, the planets will align and the tides will be in the middle of the high and low tide but as we all know, they don't stay in these states for very long.

The best we can do in regard to the ongoing dynamic movement from yin to yang, is to reduce the intensity and extremity of these shifts. So instead of having extreme yang periods of excitement, action, and intensity followed by extreme periods of fatigue, sadness, and sometimes depression is to become more steady and more in control of our thoughts, emotions, actions, and internal energies. To help clarify this, the steadier, less extreme path would look more like a kind of slower and milder oscillation between yin and yang with regular and longer periods through a balanced state. Whereas the opposed, the more extreme expressions of yin and yang, would look more like sharper, quicker, and more spikey oscillations, which include more extreme highs and lows with very quick and shorter periods passing through the balanced state.

For the human being, the wisest approach is to first accept that yin and yang are dynamic forces and there will always be movement from one to the other, with balanced states coming and going. The second thing we can do is learn to flow with it, not against it, and in doing so, recognize that this emotional state, this situation, and so on will always change. The third thing we can do is to avoid pushing ourselves to either extreme through building awareness and adjusting our lifestyles. Although mankind has little control over the yin and yang forces expressing themselves throughout the universe, man does, however, have a unique capacity to learn and adjust the behaviors that help govern the yin and yang energies playing out in our own body and mind. The general principle being that we are best to avoid extremes of yin or yang energy, if possible. Any extreme in one direction eventually triggers a dramatic shift to the opposite extreme, which commonly manifests itself as some kind of illness, which manifests as a way for the universal forces to stop us in our tracks. Other examples of manifestations of too much extreme yin or yang are mental illness, physical degeneration, toxic organ overload, and burnout. In most cases, mostly because of our yang dominated culture, it is yang that tends to reach extreme levels before a rapid shift to yin is triggered.

Many years ago, I was treating a 30 year old fit looking man who was, until recently, a very successful sports athlete. He had been recently diagnosed with chronic fatigue syndrome as he was in a great deal of pain, fatigue, and mental confusion. After speaking with him during the treatment, I discovered that he had been training and competing in sports nearly every day of his life since he was 6 or 7 years old and in all that time, he had rarely had any time off to relax and just take some time out for himself. What became obvious to me is that he had been pushing yang, yang, yang for over 20 years and he had reached the point that yang collapsed and became yin. He was now flattened, unable to walk very far, and in a great deal of discomfort. Pushing and pushing yang, or yin, for long enough and it will collapse and bring the other energy in as an attempt to bring things back to some balance. Unfortunately for this young man, he was in the middle of a tough and long journey back to health and balance. In many cases of such extremes, it can take at least a year or three, that is if the person comes to accept their current condition and is proactive in getting their health and well-being slowly, patiently, and mindfully back into place.

The feelings associated with a completely balanced state tend to be a feeling that is devoid of the pulls of desires, wants, and needs on all levels. There is a state of no cravings for any particular outcomes, no real hunger, no need for mental stimulation, and little to no interest in seeking out excitement. There is a natural and automatic experiencing of contentedness with whatever "is". *This word that best describes this experience is acceptance.* A deep feeling of acceptance permeates throughout our body and mind. Suddenly, there is a feeling of deep acceptance of one's life situation, acceptance of others, acceptance of this, acceptance of that, and even the acceptance of the world's current state, no matter how ghastly it may appear. It's as if a higher energy state comes over us and we simply just "get it". This state, depending on the person, and as illustrated above, can last from just a few minutes to many hours or even days. The more the state is experienced, the more one's awareness sensitivity the longer one tends to sit in it. This heightened state of awareness during these periods of balance provide us a great peace, wisdom, and a taste of enlightenment, yet, it is not enlightenment. This is because even though we may be experiencing balance for a short time, this experience is still bound within the realm of yin and yang. To touch real enlightenment, it is necessary to transcend the forces of yin and yang and this is something I will talk about more later in the book.

There is one major potential trap regarding the experience of balance. Those who do not fully understand the laws of change tend to become attached to the pleasurable states experienced when one touches balance. When one becomes attached to this pleasurable balanced state, a great deal of tension will arise when the balanced state dissolves and the next phase of yin or yang arises, which is inevitable. Therefore, when experiencing the pleasurable balanced state, it is essential to let the phases of yin, yang, and this balanced state to still move through us unhindered as this will allow the flow of life to continue in a fluid and healthy manner and reduce the potential of extreme oscillations.

The Yin and Yang Quiz

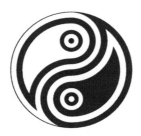

"We may be floating on Tao, but there is nothing wrong with steering. If Tao is like a river, it is certainly good to know where the rocks are." ~ Deng Ming Dao

In this chapter, we utilize a quiz that has been designed to help us identify if we are predominately running on yang energy or yin energy at this time in our lives.

We are born into this world with either a yin or yang predominate constitution, which governs the tendencies of our bodies and our minds. It is absolutely necessary to become aware of what yin and or yang quality is most influential to us so that we can be more proactive and aware as to where to focus our attention and adjust our lifestyles to support our evolution.

The results of this quiz will provide us with greater insight into our current energetic influence and help us to identify the potential influence of our constitutional nature. If, after completing the quiz, you discover that you are predominately yang in nature, then your greatest work and challenge for this lifetime is to be bringing more yin into your world and if you discover that you are predominately yin, the focus will be on cultivating more yang. You will probably find that it is the activities that promote the opposite forces to balance us out are the ones we tend to avoid and dislike the most. This is a clear indicator as to our underlying constitutional tendencies. To bring more attention on the opposite generates a more well-rounded individual, one who can handle and adapt to challenges and change more easily. Those who do not focus on working with the opposite tend to be stubborn, narrow minded, and unable to adapt to changing circumstances. What also has been found over time when working with the opposite is that what initially presents as a challenge and dislike, actually becomes an enjoyable practice, one that is recognized as a necessary and beneficial.

Below is the 10 question Yin Yang Quiz. Circle the answer that relates to you most of the time. Add up the scores at the end to receive your results. *Please note, this quiz only serves as guide and is not intended to replace the advice of a qualified health professional in a clinical setting.*

The Yin and Yang Quiz

Question	Answer	Points
1. Do you get headaches?	Never	1
	Rarely	2
	Sometimes	3
	Often	4
	Always	5
2. Do you have a thin or wiry body shape?	No	1
	Not really	3
	Yes	5
3. Do you tend to eat your food very	Very fast	5
	I finish before most people	4

fast or do you take your time and eat it slowly?	- A steady pace	3
	- Slower than most people	2
	- I'm always the last to finish	1
4. Do you find it hard to wind down, switch off and relax?	- Very hard, I often take alcohol or drugs to help calm me down	5
	- Difficult	4
	- Most of the time, it's okay	3
	- It's easy to switch off	2
	- Always relaxed and can go to sleep at any time	1
5. Do you find it easy to get to sleep and stay asleep?	- No, I find it hard to get to sleep and I wake often	5
	- No, I find it hard to get to sleep but once I get to sleep, I'm okay	4
	- Generally, yes	3
	- Most of the time, I can get to sleep easily and stay asleep	2
	- I'm always tired, I could sleep standing up	1
6. Do you consider yourself a patient person?	- No way, I become easily agitated when I have to wait for anything	5
	- Not usually, if you catch me on a good day, I'm okay	4
	- Most of the time	3
	- Yes	2
	- I don't mind waiting, I actually enjoy it	1
7. Do you find it easy to be alone and occupy yourself?	- Yes, I really enjoy being alone	1
	- Most of the time	2
	- It doesn't bother me	3
	- I prefer to be around my friends and other people	4
	- I can't stand being alone	5

8. On your weekends and holidays, do you prefer to sleep a lot and hang out at home or do you prefer to go out to different events and stay up late partying?	- Sleep a lot and stay at home, I rarely want to go out	1
	- I prefer to relax at home most of the time	2
	- I like to do both if I have the time	3
	- I prefer going out to various events and partying when I have the chance	4
	- Party every night! Boom Boom!	5
9. Are you the first person in the room to feel the cold?	- Yes, I always get cold easily	1
	- Most of the time	2
	- Not really	3
	- No, I tend to enjoy the cool	4
	- No way, I wear hardly any clothes and I'm still hot	5
10. Do you drink alcohol or coffee every day?	- Yes, at least 3 coffees or glasses of alcohol a day	5
	- Yes, under 3 coffees or glasses of alcohol a day	4
	- Not every day	3
	- Rarely	2
	- I don't drink any coffee or alcohol	1

Finished! Great, now add up all the points on your answers and go to the next page to view your results.

Results of Yin Yang Quiz

Less than 22 = Yin dominant

You tend to have more *Yin* characteristics than Yang characteristics. To establish more of a balance, it is advised to generate more energy and heat in your body by engaging with some of the following suggestions found throughout this book.

Between 22 and 28 = Balanced

You have come up as being in a relatively balanced state of Yin and Yang. It is quite a rare thing, so well done! Generally, I would say to keep doing whatever it is you are doing, you are on a good wicket. The suggestions found throughout this book will surely help you to keep you steady.

You can always take it further by committing to a more serious mediation practice because you are probably ripe for it. Remember to continue to surround yourself with natural beauty, keep the exercise going to keep your body flowing, and keep yourself connected to your passions and inspirations as they will carry you through.

Greater than 28 = Yang dominant

You tend to have more *Yang* characteristics than Yin characteristics. To establish more of a balance, it is advised to cultivate more relaxation and gentleness by engaging in some of the following suggestions found throughout this book.

Yang Lifestyle

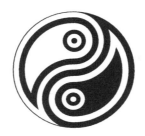

"The path to success is to take massive, determined action."
~ Anthony Robbins

This chapter is dedicated to exploring a yang dominant lifestyle. This is actually the most common tendency these days as the modern world emphasizes and encourages action, ambition, force, and excitement, which are all primarily yang in nature. Yang lifestyles also tend to be associated with extroverted personalities, as extroverts tend to gain more energy the more they interact with people and the more they busy themselves. Being yang'd up is not a bad thing or a good thing, it just is what it is. Yin and yang are neither bad nor good, they just are. Remember that yin and yang are not personal. They are just expressions of the universal forces at play.

Yang energy is extremely helpful in our world as it gets things done. It is the energy of action and of inspiration and those with a good dose of yang tend to generate wealth and business success simply because of the extra level of enthusiasm they add to life. Without a good dose of yang energy every now and then, we would become completely inactive, stagnant, passive, and uninspired. With yang energy, we get to participate in life, we get to express, progress, work, interact, build, and experience new things. Yang is what gives our world color and dynamism. With a good balance of yang energy, we are willing and enthusiastic to participate in life, to learn, grow, and evolve.

When yang energy is left to run wild for long and excessive periods of time, it can easily lead to a yang extreme, which often expresses itself as malice, aggression, violence, intolerance, and ruthlessness in thought, word, or deed. When we overdose on yang, we can easily lose control and become like a raging bush fire, burning up ourselves and harming those with whom we come into contact with. When we get to these extremes states, it is a sign we have gone too far and need to pull ourselves back toward yin energy to encourage a more balanced state. The most obvious way to do this is to first discontinue and walk away from the current activity or action that is fueling the fire. It could be a form of stimulation or circumstance that triggers yang energy to flow in excessive amounts throughout your system. The second step after walking away, is to ride out the storm by focusing on the present moment, allowing our breath to stabilize and letting our feelings and the emotions settle. A quick way to snap ourselves out of a particular harmful and over-reactive pattern is to step away and surrender the intense emotions, feelings, and thoughts over to the universe, to completely let it go. It is better to withdraw, become quiet, and wait out the storm than to keep on raging ahead with greater potential to cause harm to ourselves and to others. With enhanced awareness, we come to see what activities or situations trigger us toward such excessive states so as to empower ourselves to take wiser action in the future.

Below is a list of activities that would enhance yang energy. Remember that neither yin or yang energy are 'wrong' or 'bad', but are just expressions of natural laws.

- Alcohol
- Taking stimulants (coffee, amphetamines, tobacco, energy drinks, etc.)
- Willingness, enthusiasm
- Committing to work and setting goals
- Being busy, taking on many commitments
- Ambition and drive
- Partying
- Weight lifting, running, hot yoga, extreme sports
- Stubbornness, inflexible
- Over-planning, overthinking, over-talking
- Easy to frustration and anger
- Over-committing
- Always seeking adventure, action, doingness

Signs and symptoms of excess Yang
- Regular headaches
- Insomnia
- Thin body frame
- Finds it hard to sit still for any length of time
- Hot body temperature, easy to sweat
- Usually easy to anger or frustration
- Red face, red, blood shot eyes
- Loud voice
- Doesn't stop talking
- Cannot sit still
- Needs constant stimulation
- Hypertension
- Addictions

Signs and Symptoms of Yang in balance
- Ambitious but is still able to switch off easily (5pm onward)
- Enthusiastic, energetic but is able to relax, sit still, and sleep when the time comes.

- Regular body temperature. Warm, but not hot.
- Little to no headaches
- Patient, yet persistent
- Willing to learn and grow
- Enthusiastic about life, inspired
- Enjoys rest, work, and play
- Clear strong voice, doesn't over-speak, chooses words carefully
- Motivates and inspires others through their own passion and drive
- Regular, steady stream of energy throughout the day. No big ups and no big downs. Doesn't need to take stimulants every day
- Can sit still when the moment arises
- Is perfectly fine without stimulation

Yin Lifestyle

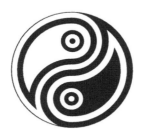

"Peace is the result of training your mind to process life as it is, rather than as you think it should be." ~ Dr. Wayne Dyer

This chapter is dedicated to exploring in more detail yin energy and how it manifests and expresses itself in human activities. The keywords for yin are relaxation, creativity, contentment, and peacefulness. Yin personalities would be associated more with introverted personalities because of their desire to be alone more often than not. However, introverts, without proper balance or healthy habits, can easily become intense, obsessive, neurotic, and mentally unstable. Therefore, practices like yoga, tai chi, or martial arts are particularly helpful for yin type personalities as it gives them a healthy channel for their energy, grounds them into their bodies, and brings them out of the intensity of their inner world. The ultimate yin expression is being able to fully relax into, and be content with, the uncertainty and movement of life.

Yin energy is often resisted and seen as boring and lacking something. This is because most humans are pumped up on yang and therefore overlook the subtler benefits yin energy provides. Another reason why it is often avoided or overlooked is because it is slower than yang energy. Yang energy is fast and gives results quickly. Yin, on the other hand, is slow and yielding, which requires more time, focus, and persistence to see the results. Yet, in the long term, we can come to see that yin, when given the chance, can be much more powerful than yang energy. Taoist sages often associate yin energy to be like water and yang to be like stone. Stone is strong in structure and form whereas water is weak in structure and form, yet, over time, water wears away stone and shapes it according to its own nature. Another example is we can see in those people who really stick to a goal or a project where many people give up and move onto other things. These people often sacrifice many other things in their lives to follow through and complete their project to the very end. And it is these people who achieve amazing and wondrous results only capable of those who remain focused and persistent on a particular goal. Those who fly in and fly out from one project to the next tend to lack the inner power developed when one develops inner yin energy.

Yin energy is what gives our world peace, relaxation, joyful presence, awareness, gratitude, wisdom, and deep appreciation. Without yin energy, we would all be running around in a mass of chaotic activity without any capacity for appreciation, enjoyment, or reflection.

Below is a list of activities that would enhance yin energy.
- Sleeping
- Resting
- Meditation
- Patient, persistent,
- Focused
- Reading books
- Not over committing oneself
- Lack of desires, lack of planning
- Slow walking, yin yoga, restorative yoga, tai chi

- Contemplation
- Easy going, flexible
- Being alone for extended periods
- Sitting still

Signs and symptoms of excess Yin
- Poor digestion
- Overweight
- No motivation, no enthusiasm
- Sinus, phlegm
- Over sleeps, lethargic
- Slow to think
- Apathy (I can't do it.. etc.)
- Passive suicide (self-destructive – poor food choices, etc.)

Signs and Symptoms of Yin predominate personality in Balance
- Curvaceous, not overweight, not underweight.
- Driven and inspiring, yet easy to relax
- Insightful, intelligent, wise
- Clear and articulate speaker
- Creative, intuitive
- Comfortable in their own space or being alone
- Easy going, relaxed, in the moment

The Modern Human Experience is Yang'd Up

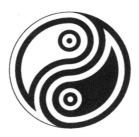

"Modern man thinks he loses something; time, when he does not do things quickly. Yet he does not know what to do with the time he gains except to kill it." ~ Eric Fromm

At this time in human and earthly evolution, the collective consciousness of humanity, as a whole, is out of balance. There is simply too much yang and not enough yin. This has been the case for the last hundreds and potentially thousands, of years, hence, the madness throughout human history with the continuous engagement in war, greed, environmental degradation, and the exploitation of other beings.

During this time in our human and planetary journey, the human consciousness evolution is slowly moving from a yang dominant state to a more yin and balanced state. This transition is largely coming about as humans become more sensitive and aware of the interconnectedness of all things. Although this is not a new idea, not many humans actually embody it, understand it, and live in accordance with it. On the intellectual level, it is easy to understand, but on the actual level, it is often very difficult to understand. Ongoing observation, meditation, and self-reflection are some of the best tools to assist in this actualization process.

Humans are slowly coming to realize our true innate connection with Mother Nature and our connection to each other and all of life. Through this understanding, we come to see the Mother Earth and each other as extended expressions of our own selves and, therefore, we do not seek to hurt or harm others because to do so creates a negative ripple throughout all of humanity, which, in turn, only harms ourselves. When we look at each other from a yang dominant state, what we see is separation and this creates the destructive "I – Me" complex. When we view ourselves as a separate "I - Me", we are free to carry out thoughts, words, and deeds with the primary aim to satisfying and uplifting the "I - Me" complex, which usually comes at the cost of other beings. There is a way to live in this world where the having and receiving does not come at the cost of taking away from another, which incites poverty, but rather, the having and receiving is of a mutual benefit, where an energetic and material exchange is in place, which benefits all beings.

As we move into the next necessary stage of the human evolution process, the cultivation of yin energy is recommended as a way to create a smoother and more graceful transition into the next stage. Those who have a cultivated a good dose of yin will be much more at ease during the next stage of our collective human evolution. Those who remain in a state of excess yang and have not worked to cultivate any yin energy will likely find it difficult over next few decades with regular and frequent experiences of anxiety, uneasiness, and agitation.

For humanity to continue to survive and thrive, I believe many of us will need to focus more intensely on cultivating the yin energy within. If we do not, as a collective, humanity will likely write its own fate toward self-destruction.

The Yin Yang Split

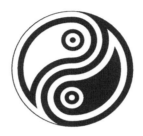

In my acupuncture and yoga teaching practice, I often see people who have what I have termed a 'yin-yang split'. It occurs when the mind and body become disconnected. The mind, mostly as a result over thinking (which often includes some kind of obsessive behavior with computer technologies), and the body becoming under stimulated (yin), creates the conditions for the energy of yin and yang to split inside the human being.

Because this splitting of yin and yang within the human being, it goes against the inner nature and, therefore, it creates a complex condition that affects humans on many levels. When the mind and body disconnect, the spirit is dislodged and confused and when ongoing, often this leads to mental delusion, instability and illness, physical body degeneration, and spiritual disassociation. The mind and body need to be connected for the mind and body to function in a healthy way as well as providing an inner environment for the spiritual aspect of our natures to abide in safety. Therefore, when the mind and body are split, all spiritual guidance is greatly impaired and the human will tend to take on a very confused, scattered, and lost demeanor.

From my experience, the best thing to re-link the mind and body connection is to practice 'movement with breath'. Slow graceful movements with breath synchronizations assist in reconnecting the nervous and energetic system. For example, Qi Gong, Tai Chi, and some forms of yoga are ideal for this practice. It is often hard for some people to learn how to move slower with breath awareness, because many people have movement style patterns and behaviours well engrained in their nervous and musculoskeletal system, making it an often long and difficult process to unlearn these well established unhealthy movement patterns.

It can be as simple as practicing your preferred set of Qi Gong or yoga movements with your full attention and focus for 5-10 minutes twice a day to help to reconnect the mind and the body.

As we continue to develop greater awareness of our inner state, we can come to recognize more easily when we have spent enough time doing a particular activity. Stress signals such as digestion problems, any feelings of nausea, eye problems, and a stiffening of the neck and body are all signs that the mind and body are under stress and beginning to disconnect. When we sense our bodies and minds beginning to disconnect from each other, we need to take necessary action to avoid this from becoming too excessive, which is usually as simple as stepping away from your computer or activity, taking a drink of water, and stepping outside for 5 minutes to stretch and relax. During these 'break times', avoid loud music or TV's because they fill up the space and impair your nervous system and energetic system the ability to settle and reorganise. Just observe. Feel your body, feel the sensations, allow your breath to settle, and stretch a little. Just be with it and wait a little while. When you wait long enough, nature will make it obvious when it is time to return to your project.

The Yin and Yang of Clock Time

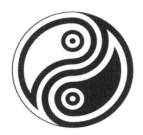

Throughout a 24 hour daily cycle, yin and yang play a very powerful influence in the overall energy throughout the day. It is helpful to become aware of how yin and yang flow throughout the day so that we can orientate our work and lifestyle to align with these forces. Aligning with them brings about greater fluidity in our work, relationships, and our creativity.

Below is an outline of the 24hr cycle and how yin and yang play out.

12 midnight – 3am
This phase of time is the peak of Yin energy. The night sky is at its darkest and within the human realm, the dream state is at its deepest. Every night, when we experience deep sleep, we have the opportunity to shed the limitations of the physical body. We are allowed to play and explore the universe in our purely energetic body. It is during these deep sleep states that we are more open and receptive to receive various teachings and information from the universe that can be used to help us in our evolution. Many messages we receive are also provided to us so that we are then guided in our daily physical world experience.

As well as dreaming during this time, our physical bodies are given the perfect opportunity to rest, digest, and repair. Our bodies go into a kind of restoration mode that naturally cultivates yin energy throughout our being.

If we suffer from insomnia, irregular sleeping patterns, or light sleep, we do not have the opportunity to repair our bodies or receive guiding messages from the dream world. Short periods that consist of only a few days of sleep disturbance tend to be a natural part of the human experience and are, therefore, nothing to worry about as healthy sleep will surely return after a few days have passed. It is the long term, chronic sleep disturbance patterns that really need to be corrected if we are to have any chance of reducing extreme expressions of yin and yang in our lives. Healthy sleep patterns come from working with yin and yang during our awake, conscious daily life. Meditation, hypnosis, binaural beats, magnesium supplements, psychotherapy, acupuncture, yoga, and reducing yang style activities will all assist in restoring healthy sleeping habits.

3am – 6am

Yin is dominant, yet yang is starting to rise. This is a good time to get up and out of bed, getting ready for the day. Exercising and doing some physical training (yoga, martial arts, tai chi, etc.) at this time is actually the most beneficial time for the body and the energetic systems. The yin of night comes to a close as yang starts to rise.

This is also a good time for meditation practice because this time provides a window where yin and yang are in transition. It is as if yang energy is waking up and sending out a giant cosmic wave of energy. Thus, meditating and giving attention to our affirmations during this time will help us to ride the cosmic yang wave and utilize its power.

6am – 9am

Yang continues to rise, gaining more and more momentum. This is the best time to eat a grounding and nutritious breakfast with plenty of proteins to set you up for the day ahead. After we fill our bellies and cells with food energy, it time to set ourselves up for our becoming stuck into our work life flow. Around 9am is the best time to start digging in.

9am – 12midday

Yang is rising and starting to peak. This is the best time to focus on your toughest thinking tasks and tackle them head on. This is the most productive time for working and thinking that includes facing and addressing any difficult customers or clients. Naturally, earlier in the day tends to be a lot less emotional so it's a good time to face those difficult clients or talk over difficult subjects with colleagues or partners. It's important not to waste this time of the day, in regard to your workflow and productivity.

12midday – 3pm

Yang is peaking. After your intense work phase earlier on, it now time to back off a bit and take the time to eat a nourishing, protein packed lunch. Because of the extra yang energy in the environment, the digestive system is at its peak and therefore, it tends to be able to handle larger portions of food, but this does not mean overeating, which often makes people feel tired and sluggish for the rest of the day. Around lunch time is also the best time to meetings and discuss grand ideas for the future of projects. Why not meet up with a colleague over lunch and discuss the future visions and inspirational ideas you have. Let the yang of the day motivate, inspire, and move you at this time. After lunch, it's good to back off your intensity a bit, allowing yourself to have a little rest, time out, or even a 20 minute nap. After your lunch and little rest, it's time to get back but with less intensity then in the morning as yin is starting to creep its way back in. As the afternoon comes around, this time is much more suited to doing simpler tasks like replying to easy emails and tying up any loose ends. You may even want to focus more on the creative aspects of your work to lighten things up a bit and make it more fun.

3pm – 6pm
Yang has peaked out and now yin is now beginning to descend. As the afternoon and evening come closer, yin invites us to really slow down, and start wrapping up any serious work related activities. Around 5, it's a great time to clock out, change your clothes, have a shower, and relax into the night ahead.

6pm – 9pm
Yin is well and truly present. The sun has disappeared over the horizon and the stars are glistening in the night sky. This is one of the most creative times of the 24hr cycle because yin is associated with relaxation and creativity. Working on some creative project that helps you relax, having sex, and listening to your favorite music is ideal at this time. Watching a little TV is fine, too, if it helps you laugh, relax, and switch off of work mode. Best to avoid commercial TV or the news as this tends to cause stress to our system. Between 6pm and 9pm, think of this time as a safe time to reconnect with your creativity and have a bit of relaxed fun. During this time, give yourself permission to let go of the troubles of the day, knowing that you can deal with them tomorrow morning if need be. When we can approach bed time with a sense of warmth and relaxation, sleep comes easily, joyfully, and pleasantly.

9pm – 12midnight

Yin energy has fully descended and is soon to reach its peak. It is time to withdraw from the activities of the world and enter into our sleep and dream state. This period in time provides us with another doorway from the activities of the world and into the depth of the energetic dream world. It is advised to be in bed before 11pm at the latest, because to stay up any longer can often lead to missing this yin energetic doorway that opens into the inner being and dream world. It can be helpful to sit quietly for a few minutes just before bed to reflect upon your day, to see if there are things that you learned, and things you could do better. If there is any intense emotional energy present before you go to bed, it is advisable to sit quietly in meditation until your breath stabilizes and the energy dissipates.

The Yin and Yang of Food

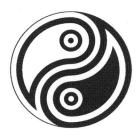

"To keep our body healthy is a duty, otherwise we shall not be able to keep our mind strong and clear." ~ Buddha

Yang = Hot, Spicy, Acidic
Yin = Cold, Raw, Alkaline

In Oriental culture, the theory of yin and yang in relation to food has been thoroughly investigated and practiced throughout the ages. For thousands of years, the ancient Chinese observed the actions of food on our bodies and our minds. They were able to distinguish which foods were more yang in nature and which foods were more yin. The most basic principle of the yin and yang of food is found with the essential heating nature of food. If it is hot, as in spicy hot, it is considered yang. If it is cooling, it is considered yang. Disease in the human body often manifests as what they consider either a hot disease or a cold disease. Hot disease is found when the patient suffers from a fever and elevated body temperature. So, in many cases, if such a disease presented, a prescription of yin energy cooling foods would be administered for healing as well as nutritional support. In cases of a disease that brings coldness throughout the body and a colder body temperature, yang energy heating foods would be administered.

It is important to note that the body is around the average temperature of 38° Celsius and in most cases, is slightly hotter than the environmental temperature of the external environment. Therefore, to have slightly warm foods is generally considered to be "neutral" because the body's natural state to be slightly warm.

Here is a list of foods that have been split up into their various states of yin or yang. Depending on your reference material and the cultural context, some foods can be found to vary in their yin or yang categorization. This list, therefore, aims to serve only as a guide.

General Foods

Very Yin	Yin	Neutral	Yang	Very Yang
Aloe Vera	Apple	Almond	Alcohol	Strong Alcohol
Asparagus	Alfalfa	Aduki Beans	Astragalus	Chilly
Avocado	Banana	Butter	Black beans	Pepper
Seaweed	Beetroot	Carrot	Bay leaf	Ginger
Cashew	Cabbage	Eggs	Cardamom	Garlic
Cucumber	Celery	Corn	Cauliflower	Cinnamon
Grapefruit	Cream	Ginko	Coffee	
Ice cream	Green Tea	Lentil	Coriander	
Kelp	Melon	Liquorish	Dill	
Kiwi Fruit	Lemon	Maize	Fennel	
Lotus Root	Lettuce	Malt	Frankincense	
Mung Bean	Lime	Cow milk	Ginseng	
Seaweed	Linseed	Rice milk	Guava	

Pear Juice	Mango	Miso	Horseradish	
Rhubarb	Milk soy	Mushroom	Jasmine	
Salt	Mulberry	Oats	Lamb	
Soy sauce	Orange	Olive	Leek	
Sugarcane	Peppermint	Peanut	Milk goat	
Tomato	Plum	Pineapple	Mugwort	
Watermelon	Radish	Polenta	Mustard Seed	
Wheat bran	Sage	Potato	Onion	
Wolfberry	Sesame Oil	Quinoa	Oregano	
Yogurt	Spinach	Rice	Paprika	
	Tofu	Rye	Parsley	
	Watercress	Salmon	Peach	
	Wheat	Sardine	Pumpkin	
	White Wine	Turkey	Red Wine	
	Zucchini	Vanilla	Salami	
		Yam	Shallot	

The style of cooking is also considered to influence the yin and yang properties of foods. For example, to bake or cook food over an open flame is considered to be a very yang, hot style of cooking, which, in effect, will add more yang energy to the food. To steam or lightly boil food is considered a gentler way of cooking and, therefore, is considered to be less yang. Therefore, this method would be recommended for those people who tend to have too much yang in their system.

Raw foods are generally considered to be very yin and cold in nature because of the lack of exposure to any yang style cooking. Also, raw foods can often lack hot spices and heat inducing herbs that would bring the food at least up to a neutral warming state for the body. Therefore, in oriental cultures and oriental traditional medicines, raw foods are rarely used or prescribed especially in any case of disease that is presenting cold signs and symptoms. In summer and the hotter months of the year, raw and lighter foods are considered beneficial because of the excessive yang in the atmosphere. However, during winter or the cooler months, it is advised to completely steer clear of cold yin style foods.

The other consideration, in regard to food and the nature of yin and yang, is to do with acidity and alkalinity of foods. Acidity refers to foods or substances that have a pH level of 7 or less. Alkalinity refers to those foods or substances that have a pH level of 7 or over. An alkaline environment is like being in the middle of a green, luscious rainforest. The air and water is clean and pure and the environment is alive and buzzing with life. An acidic environment is more like being in the centre of a big city. The air is full of petrochemicals, the water has been processed and recycled, the roads and sidewalks are covered in grime and life struggles to survive. A highly acidic environment within our bodies encourages degeneration of tissues, illness, inflammation, and cancer. An alkaline environment in our bodies promotes cellular regeneration, good circulation and elimination, oxygenated blood, healthy tissues, and happy organs.
The ideal pH level for the average human being is slightly alkaline at 7.3-7.45. You can easily get your body's pH level by using a piece of litmus paper in your saliva or urine first thing in the morning.

Generally, it has been well accepted in the world of modern day nutrition that alkaline based foods are more acceptable and beneficial for health than acidic foods. The general recommendation lays somewhere around 70-80% alkaline food and 20-30% acidic for ideal nutritional health.
For most people in the western world, however, it has been found that diets mainly consist of acidic foods more so then alkaline

foods, which, over time, often gives rise and contributes to various diseases, inflammatory conditions, and degenerative conditions. Although this is not a new concept and understanding into the field of nutritional science, it is still not well known or practiced because of the medical field's slow acceptance to acknowledge that nutrition does in fact play a big part in someone's overall physical and mental health.

The Yin and Yang of Coffee

It only takes a morning stroll down an inner city street to see an abundance people lining the sidewalks of their favorite coffee shops, hankering out for their morning coffee hit. Coffee could well be considered the life blood of our modernized yang dominated civilization because coffee in essence, because of its stimulating effect on our system, is yang energy.

Because of our current obsession with coffee, I thought it appropriate to explore a variety of coffee drinks to help uncover what coffee drinks produce the most yang effect and what produces the most subdued, more yin type effects.

As a general rule of thumb, milk is a yin substance because it is cold, wet, and phlegmy and results in a cooling effect on the body. The more milk products we add to a coffee, the more yin it becomes.

Espresso/Short Black
- Short hit of water and black coffee – very yang

Double espresso
- Double hit of water and black coffee – very, very yang

The Americano
- One shot of coffee with extra water – yang

Café latte
- One shot of coffee with milk and milk froth – yang with a large dose of yin

Cappuccino
- One shot of coffee with milk and lots of milk froth – yang with a good dose of yin

Café mocha
- One shot of coffee with milk, milk froth, and chocolate syrup – mainly yang with some yin

Flat white
- One shot of coffee with milk, no froth – yang with yin

Macchiato
- Short black with a little milk froth – very yang with a tiny bit of yin

Iced coffee (little milk)
- One shot of coffee with milk and ice - slightly yang with a large dose of yin

Iced coffee with cream, ice cream, and added flavors
- One shot of coffee with lots of milk, cream, ice cream, and ice - mostly yin with a tiny bit of yang

Hot milk (no coffee)
- no coffee shot, just warmed up milk – very yin

The Yin and Yang of Exercise

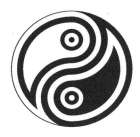

"Never limit where running can take you. I mean geographically, spiritually and of course physically." ~ *Bart Yasso*

Yang = fast, repetitive movements, heavy, intense
Yin = slower, deeper, suspended holds, light, gentle

The premise to all exercise, whether we are aware of it or not, is to apply varied amounts of stress and damage on the tissues of the body (mainly muscle tissue) so that the body repairs and regenerates itself to be bigger and better than before the stress was applied. This is why, after a good workout, we often feel sore the next day or for a few days afterward. The soreness of the muscles are because of damaged tissues and fibers, which, over the next few days, will repair and in doing so, the aches and pains will dwindle away, leaving us feeling stronger and more able than before. Therefore, when we are going to do some exercise, what we are really saying is that we are going to apply stress to the body's tissues so that they will repair themselves in a stronger and improved state.

The opposite of exercise is to live a very sedentary existence, where no stress is applied to any of the tissues of the body. What happens in this case is that the muscles and tissues begin to breakdown into a state of atrophy, which, in turn, weakens the fibers and tissues and leaves us with less strength, less flexibility, and with less energy overall.

Therefore, as long as we have a human body, we need to apply ongoing, regular, mild to moderate amounts of stress to it to keep it in a healthy, functioning, strong, and energized state. Too much exercise and the tissues can be injured and too little exercise and the body deteriorates.

In the world of exercise, yang exercise can be defined as those movements and actions that tend to be quick, intense, and repetitive. This approach to exercise can be seen in gyms all throughout the world. These kinds of actions produce a great deal of heat and perspiration, which is what most people are striving for when they apply themselves to exercise. We have all become so accustomed to this approach to exercise that many of us have never stopped to ponder it. We associate these fast and intense movements, which generate a lot of heat and perspiration, to be doing something of value and, therefore, any movement or action that is not of this nature is not considered to be exercise.

Although yang based movements are an essential part of exercise as a whole, what is often overlooked is the more yin aspects of exercise. Yin style exercise involves moving in a way that generates a sense of yielding and mindfulness within an action. It usually involves moving much slower, using longer sustainable holds, and the deliberate placement of attention to various parts of the body or mind. Two of the best examples to help illustrate this more yin approach to exercise are Qi Gong and restorative yoga. Even though these forms are not focused on quick movements, they yield powerful effects on the body and mind. Practicing mindful attention placement enhances the effects of any exercise because it connects the body (yin) to the mind (yang). When these two are united, a great deal of extra power becomes available via the forces of yin and yang. Another important aspect that yin exercises have to offer is that they work on tissues of the body that are not able to be deeply accessed in yang exercise. There a masses amounts of connective tissue around the joints, bones, organs, and muscles. Connective tissue is like a plastic wrapper that surrounds and connects everything throughout the body. The unique thing about connective tissue is that it takes time to yield and lengthen. When muscle fibers are active, the deeper connective tissue layers are inaccessible because the muscles are holding and pulling things together. Therefore, to reach these deeper layers, we need to hold stretches, without any muscle activation, for at least 2-3 minutes. Musculoskeletal medical conditions such as fibromyalgia, I believe is mainly the result of the connective tissue being tight probably because the deeper layers of it have never been fully lengthened. We are also discovering that stress factors influence this connective tissue, which cause it to tighten. When connective tissue tightens, it has the potential to tighten around everything, the heart, the brain, the joints, the organs, and so on. So if we really want to approach exercise in a balanced and supportive way, we really have to take the time to work with both yin and yang styles of exercise.

Injuries often occur during exercise in those exercise style program that encourage intense, mindless practice (mindless practice refers to exercise where there is no importance placed on awareness of body or mind, which is another contributing factor toward a yin yang split complex mentioned in an earlier chapter). Many people, although with good intentions, tend to literally throw their bodies like ragdolls into rigorous and inefficient movements, which often leads to injury and the re-affirming of poor movement behaviours. Injuries often occur, which puts a sudden and sometimes painful stop to their exercise program and can even emotionally turn people off exercising all together.

Exercising in this way is often seen by many to be really hard work, really hard and really painful. This attitude comes about because we have not learnt the intelligent way to exercise. Intelligent exercise involves being aware of both the yin and yang aspects of exercise and, therefore, trains efficiently, effectively, mindfully, and joyfully.

A beneficial approach to exercise during the initial stages is to go in gradually and build up slowly toward a stronger practice. Focus must be given to warming up the joints, stretching the major areas of the body with sustained holds of at least 30 seconds to 3 minutes (for long holds, use props to help support your body so that you're not stressing out your joints), and developing the skills of mindful, attention focused movements (e.g., Not watching TV during exercise periods) so as to assist the nervous system and body to adjust and integrate.

The nervous system takes time to establish new neural pathways in the brain and nervous system, and for this occur in the most efficient ways is to not cause too much stress on our system. You cause stress whenever you push your body to 100% or beyond. When you push this hard your nervous system has no time and space to adjust and adapt. Therefore, especially when starting out with any new exercise or movement, it is advisable to go to a maximum of 80% of your capacity for the first few times so that it doesn't shock your system and stress your joints too much. After a few times repeating the movements, your nervous system will be well adjusted and then you can then move up to the 90-100% range to increase the yang potential of the exercise. However, whenever you add a new movement pattern into your training, return to 80% of your capacity until your system has adjusted to it. Training in this way is the smart use of both yin and yang energies and will only help to enhance yang style training.

When engaging in exercises and exercise programs, it is important to consider the other aspects of lifestyle that support exercise, in particular, the diet and the time of day you have dedicated to exercise. A diet that consists of a good balance of yin (alkaline) and yang (acidic) foods will enhance exercise results. More about diet is mentioned in another chapter. Intense, more yang styles of exercise (weights, running, etc.) are more suited to the mornings and middle of the day, whereas the evenings are more suited to yin style exercises like stretching, walking, and gentle movements (yoga, tai chi, etc.).

The Yin and Yang of Yoga

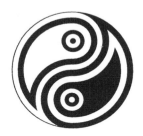

"To perform every action artfully is yoga." ~ *Swami Kripalu*

Yang = strong, active, repetitive, muscular, Rajas
Yin = gentler, meditative, suspended movements, connective tissue, Tamas

Within the yoga world of today, there is a style of yoga known as yin yoga and its primary focus and teaching is on the connective tissues of the body. Although this is true in relation to its particular context, that being of comparing muscle tissue to connective tissue, we can shift the context to address slightly different approach. For the purpose of this book, and to help us gain deeper and thorough understandings of yin and yang, let's look at yoga more so as a strong, stimulating style practice that we call yang yoga and a slower, deeper, and more meditative practice which may be referred to as yin yoga. This means that we shall leave the whole focus on the tissues of the body and anatomy elements out of it. What we want to explore here is the energetic essence of yoga and whether it serves to stimulate a yang state or and yin state.

Stronger yoga styles like ashtanga, vinyasa, Hot yoga, and power yoga are all primarily yang style of yoga as they are more focused on generating immense amounts of heat in the body.

Slower and gentler styles of yoga such as restorative yoga, yin yoga, and gentle yoga are focused more on the slowing down of the body movements and enhancing awareness and mindfulness, and are considered to be more yin in nature.

If you are interested in yoga and yoga practice, it's important to consider whether a yang style practice or a yin style practice may be more suitable for you. Generally speaking, and contrary to what many studios would have you think, yang yoga is not good for everyone and, in some cases I have seen, stressed out anxious types of people tend to practice a lot of yang style yoga. Many times, these people attend a yang yoga class and come out at the end of it still agitated and highly strung simply because many yang styles of yoga are very stimulating and fast paced, which means your mind has to be very quick to keep up. For these people, I would say that yin styles of yoga would be much more beneficial to help them slow down. For those who already have a lot of heat in their bodies, who have hypertension, high stress levels, have trouble sleeping, and are easily agitated and on edge, yang yoga, in my opinion, is not recommended.

Likewise, those who are very yin in nature would benefit more from a yang style yoga practice as it would greatly help them to stimulate their dormant energy potential and help to stimulate their metabolism and circulation. Yang style yoga is great for those who feel stagnant or have a tendency toward depression because both of these symptoms are typical signs that energy is stuck in the body, waiting to be activated. Yang helps us to activate and switch on our nervous system, which can easily snap us out of unhelpful headspaces and negative attitudes.

When you are new to the yoga journey, it is best to explore lots of different styles (both yin and yang), different studios, and different teachers before you settle into one particular style. It will also help greatly to take into consideration whether you are predominantly yin or yang in nature so you know what area to work on first. When you find a style, a studio, and a teacher that really "clicks" with you, then to gain the most benefit, you really need to commit to a practice for at least 6-12 months. During this period, do not become distracted by the other styles and teachings. It's important to become established and grounded in one particular style first as this will lay your foundations for the future. After this period, you will probably be drawn to explore the other teachings but during that initial 6-12 month stage, don't let yourself waver or you'll be moving from one thing to the other without actually getting any real depth out of any of it.

Yoga builds strength, improves balance, and increases flexibility. However, what I have found is that it does not necessarily improve cardiovascular health as much as we would like to believe. Sure, it stimulates heart rate and gets people to sweat every now and then, but generally, the heart rate is not elevated for long enough periods to make any real lasting impact on cardiovascular fitness. Therefore, another fitness or sporting activity such as swimming, jogging, or cycling is also required alongside yoga if you wish to improve all areas of your fitness. Because the fact that yoga does not improve cardiovascular fitness in any sizable way, using it alone as a way to lose weight is not ideal. Yoga does support the process of weight loss because of the stimulation of digestion, the increase of metabolism, and the flushing of waste in the tissues. However, for more complete and rapid weight loss, another activity that focuses on cardio fitness is advised.

The Yin and Yang of Business

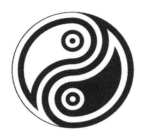

"Talk doesn't cook rice."
~ Chinese proverb

Yang = ambitious, directed, driven, action orientated, confident, growth, expanding, debt
Yin = patient, persistent, receptive, creative, relaxed, innovative, flexible, adaptable, present, credit

The business world offers us a perfect example of a yang dominated industry where ambition, action, and drive with the constant focus on growth and expansion are seen as the main elements of a successful business life. In many cases, business has become such a powerful force in our modern world that it is the accumulation of wealth through business relations and capitalist philosophy that has positioned itself as a major influence upon governments and culture. Because the business world has such a large influence on the world we live in, it is worthy of further exploration in terms of yin and yang.

Although the energy of yang is an obvious match to the activities of the business world, it's worth stepping back to consider how yin energy fits into it. We cannot ignore yin, because yin is present in some way or another, so how does it express itself in the business world, how can it help us do business in a more balanced way, and can yin actually increase productivity and business effectiveness?

Yin, in the business world, refers to the creative and innovative process. Without offering innovative and creative solutions, we don't have a business of any real value. Therefore, all valuable business ideas originally come from the creative energy of yin. Once the idea is hatched, yang energy is then required to help formulate, organize, manage, and bring the idea into the physical world through action. A lot of people tend to either have 1,000 great business ideas that are valuable, but they lack the yang energy to actualize it into reality, or people have a lot of yang energy to work on business related projects, but the ideas are lacking creative solutions and, therefore, are of no value. Without the ability to work with both yin and yang energies at the required times, it would be difficult to build any real success in the business world.

Fortunately, there are a number of strategies that can help harness these energies more effectively. One strategy is to team up with someone who helps to balance your energy. One of you may be better at digging into the details and putting things into action whereas the other may be better at coming up with the big ideas and intuiting the market. Sometimes, finding another person who has the time, drive, and interest you do is not always easy, so, in such a case, another strategy involves working on yourself. Take the time to sit down and really become clear about your strengths and supposed weaknesses. Also, become clear about your knowledge regarding the business idea you may or may not have yet and ask some important questions like: Does my idea really solve a problem and help people? Do I have enough understanding of the market that I am intending to service and work in? Do I have enough knowledge regarding the setting up and operation of a small business? If you are not able to answer these questions with a "yes", then it's time to get clued up before investing too much of your time and money. Read up on some industry web sites and check out the latest books on each of these subjects. Also, go to industry conferences and arrange appointments to talk with people you know and trust, who are connected to the industry and who could help guide you in your business idea. Of course, the actual experience and practice of running your business is where you will learn the most so be sure not to become stuck in the yin stage of just thinking, reading, and talking about it. You will eventually have to get in and take action at some stage.

The third strategy is to skill yourself up in those areas where you are lacking. Identify what skills you will require and start training yourself to get your business going or take it to the next level. With the facility of the Internet, YouTube videos, and many other sources of information, with a little investigation, it is not hard to find what information and skills you will need to skill up in the areas you have identified. The human nervous system is capable of extraordinary things and there is no limitation as to what we can train it to do. Each skill you acquire makes you, as an individual, more valuable in the marketplace and will also enable you to become flexible and adaptable as markets and industries shift over time. The trick is to never to stop learning and to keep challenging yourself while also allowing your business to innovate. If you become too complacent in the business world, the market will eventually shift and you will be left behind, allowing the opportunity for another businesses to take your place.

Going into running your own business (or contracting out your skills) is one of the most rewarding and empowering things you can do. It gives you the chance to be creative and harness your passions in a way that serves humanity and makes you money in the process. However, staying in the business game requires both the application of both yin and yang energies to be successful and to be sustainable. Action without creative thought will lead to ruin and creative thought without action will lead to stagnation and confusion.

In regard to running and managing yourself and your business, the following points will help you to identify if the business may be in need of some yin or yang energy.

The following qualities and activities are predominantly expressions of yang energy.
Are you and your business able to:
- Follow through with sales and promises to clients and industry
- Meet deadlines
- Make firm decisions when needed (e.g., Hiring, firing)
- Set goals and follow them through to completion
- Network effectively
- Willing to stand up and push out of comfort zone
- Handle late nights and early mornings
- Sacrifice other aspects of life
- Stay informed and up to date with industry
- Able to grow, expand, and increase net income
- Take risks

The following qualities and activities are predominantly expressions of yin energy.
Are you and your business able to:
- Brainstorm and share ideas regularly
- Able to innovate and adapt easily
- Listen effectively to customers' feedback

- Have periods of "stepping back" so as to gain space and contemplate the next move
- Be intuitive, which means to be open to making decisions out of intuition rather than what others advise or say
- Spend some time alone (giving staff time away to refresh)
- Grow in a steady and sustainable way
- Be patient and wait for the market to adjust itself
- Contemplate the deeper reasons for doing business (enjoyment, to serve, to help)

Another expression of yin and yang in the business and money world is yang expressed as debt and yin expressed as having real cash or credit. Debt tends to lock us up into the larger financial systems, which are heavily dependent on governments, banks, and other economic forces to keep things financially steady. When we place a lot of dependence on these systems, we are giving up a lot of our power because we are hoping that those outside system will keep our money safe. Therefore, debt tends to take away our power, which generates the feeling of lack while also causing extra stress and anxiety. Yin refers to real cash or credit, meaning we have real money available to us and, therefore, we are not so dependent on other outside forces to govern our money. When we have real cash or credit, we have power to choose what to do with our money; however, when we have debt, we have little choice as to what we can do with it. Therefore, debt creates a stressful, out of balance yang state whereas credit produces a more calming and in control yin state.

The Yin and Yang of Relaxation and Stress

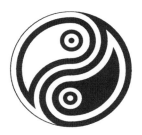

"Doing nothing is better than being busy doing nothing."
~ Lao Tzu

Yang = sympathetic nervous system, fight or flight, stress, on edge, adrenaline
Yin = parasympathetic nervous system, rest and digest, repair, relaxation

When it comes to stress and relaxation, because of their obvious natures, stress would be classified as yang energy and relaxation as yin energy. When we look at biological physiology, the nervous system operates two primary modes. One is the sympathetic nervous system mode, which is the state commonly referred to as "fight or flight" or yang energy. The other mode is the activation of the parasympathetic nervous system, which is the less well known of the two, referred to as "rest and digest" or yin energy.

In the "fight or flight" mode, the nervous system instructs the body to send a majority of its blood and energy into the extremities and muscles so that the body experiences hyper response. This is a natural part of our animal nature and it is in no way wrong for us to be triggered into this state; however, it causes us problems when we are triggered into this state for extended periods of time. Being in "flight or flight" mode for extended periods can tax our other systems and impair the whole organisms capacity to rest, rebalance, and regenerate. What also happens during the flight or flight mode is that all messages and information received through the senses are sent straight to the amygdala portion of the brain. The amygdala is a small part of brain tissue that acts like a small processor designed to trigger very basic fight or fight responses. When the amygdala is activated, the other aspects of the brain, which includes the frontal lobe, which governs the more sophisticated processing areas of the brain, are switched off. The switching off of the frontal lobe inhibits our brain's capacity to manage incoming information with greater logic, reason, and emotional capacities, therefore, limiting our ability to respond to stimulus to only that of basic primary functions. The amygdala acts as a kind of emergency processor during times of stress, which assists the nervous system to reserve energy and respond as quickly as possible. Although this is of great service when we are actually under threat, it is of no help when we are in a situations where there is no real threat and when we are trying to make a serious decisions, learn a new skill, or respond with emotional intelligence. It appears that our modern day hustle-bustle lifestyles are actually triggering this "flight or flight" amygdala brain response much more than we are aware. Common signs of being in this mode are ongoing states of anxiety, unable to sit still, unable to relax, hypertension, insomnia, rapid heart beat, or easy to anger and violent behavior.

In the other mode, we have the parasympathetic nervous system, which is dictates our "rest and digest" function. In this mode, our bodies draw energy and blood into the organs and deeper tissues for repair, support, and digestion. Our brains and nervous system also become more relaxed, which brings our breathing and heart rate down to a slower and steadier pace. A relaxed state also gives rise to enhanced mental, physical, and emotional function, resulting in being able to make better decisions, to communicate more clearly, learn better, as well as potentially enhancing our physical coordination. Naturally, we also tend to be more intuitive and creative in our work and personal life with greater potential for breakthroughs in our work and creative life. Have you ever gone to bed with a problem you just can't solve and in the morning when you wake up, the answer just appears? This is what tends to happen when we settle into yin energy of the "rest and digest" mode. In this state, the body does not tire, instead, it rests, regenerates, and repairs itself.

What I have discovered is that most people, especially those living in a fast paced modern world, are operating in the "fight or flight" mode for extended periods and are not in the "rest and digest" state long enough. What tends to happen to those who are not accessing the "rest and digest" state often enough is that they become hypertensive, stressed easily, agitated, have disturbed sleeping patterns, and may be inclined toward violence. If this goes on for long enough, eventually some kind of disease or health condition manifests, which can serve as a major warning. Those who get the message, tend to make positive and dramatic changes in the way they choose to live, often shifting their diet, exercise, work, and relationships for the better. However, those who do not heed the warning and choose not to apply any changes to their lifestyle can be expressed as yang adding to yang, which, according the natural law of yin and yang, will only lead toward disaster.

As we grow up into adulthood, many of us forget what relaxation really is and what it feels like. Many would say watching a movie and drinking a beer is relaxing, yet when we look into the physiology of these activities, we may discover that the relaxation mode is not always triggered during these activities. One reason being that many movies are full of fast flickering images, violence, and sounds designed to trigger adrenaline, designed to trigger the fight or flight response. The reason these adrenaline responses are targeted by moviemakers, TV producers, and advertising companies is because the initial rush of energy from adrenaline is generally addictive and associated with feelings of excitement. Unfortunately, the continuous focus on triggering adrenaline in people only encourages the prolonged and over-activation of the fight or flight state in people.

So, as adults, many of us have to re-learn or learn (some of us may have never known true relaxation) what true relaxation is and what it feels like. In simple descriptive language, relaxation can be described as spacious, slow, feeling satisfied, content, and a deep sense of release and calmness.

The ideal situation for a human on a biological level is to predominantly occupy the rest and digest state with the very occasional movement and oscillation into the fight or flight mode. When this is the case, sickness tends to heal more quickly and more easily, relationships are more supportive and healthy, intuition is more strongly developed, and an overall appreciation for life is greatly enhanced.

So the question arises, how does one train oneself to be more in the rest and digest state more? Later in the book, I will suggest a number of ways to bring more yin in, but for now, let's list a few here to get us started.

- Take a few conscious slow breaths in-between tasks throughout your day to bring more space and relaxation in.

- When tired, sleep. When hungry, eat. When walking, walk. When working, work. Do one thing at a time and avoid adding excess stimulation to any given task. This will increase your concentration and help you to do things more completely and with greater awareness.

- Attend gentle yoga classes.

- Learn to breathe better. The biggest tip is, when not speaking, talking, or eating, rest the tip of the tongue on the top of the mouth and breathe through your nose. Allow your breath to be smooth and steady, focusing more on a long, deep exhale breath, which helps to calm the nervous system.

- Avoid violent TV shows, violent movies, violent games, and angry sounding music. These things switch us into fight or flight mode very quickly.

- Surround yourself with natural beauty. Spend more time in nature.

- Early in the morning, practice yoga, meditation, or go for a gentle walk (with minimal talking). The morning is the best time to connect to the stillness and quiet of the day. If you do this often, you will soon notice a big shift in your energy levels and overall well-being.

- Instead of emphasizing doingness, focus on your beingness. Simply sit without doing anything for a few minutes each day. You can let the mind do its thing but just become the watcher and let it happen without becoming involved.

- Avoid filling up your spare time with more and more activities. Always allow for some space in your life where there is no plan or agenda.

The Yin and Yang of Creativity

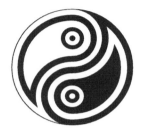

"I have never made one of my discoveries through the process of rational thinking." ~ *Albert Einstein*

Yang = action, motivation, movement, color, intensity of focus
Yin = contemplation, patience, non-movement, stepping away

The creative process is an interesting and mysterious subject, so much so that such a topic could deserve a whole book dedicated to it. Creativity, as we are all familiar with, is not a linear, step by step, rational process as a lot of other things in our lives tend to be. Creativity, like the flow of yin and yang, comes and goes. If you're lucky, it is there when you need it, but it is often not there when you need it most. The yang of creativity would refer to the actual act of doing it, of writing that book, of painting that canvas, of designing that graphic, and so on. Yang provides us with the energy to put our visions and ideas into some tangible form to bring it into the world.

What you may find, and what I have observed time and time again, is that during the initial stages of any creative project, there is plenty of yin (inspiration) and yang (doingness) available so we thrust ourselves into the project full steam. After a while, however, the energy of inspiration tends to fade and we are left with a giant task we have started out on and are now beginning to doubt if we can actually finish it. In such times, be comforted by the fact that this is a natural part of the creation process. Inspiration tends to come and go like the seasons, so it's easy and great to jump on board when it's there, but what do we do with ourselves when it fades away? In most cases, I have found and observed that it is worth continuing to work on the yang energy, which means to keep chipping away at it. Just keep digging into it, day in and day out. You can always take a moment to revisit the original inspiration that got you going in the first place, if you need a little boost. What tends to happen when you work in such a way is that eventually the inspiration will rise up again and come through reaffirming the work you have done. If you were to work on your projects only when you were inspired, it would take a very long time to complete or you would never actually finish it to the end. Yin is the capacity to have inspiration and vision whereas yang is the capacity to put it into real world action and complete it to the end.

In the creative process, yin is the primary driving force and it is the yang that brings it out of us. Yin provides us with the insight, the vision, the dream, and the idea to express ourselves and to potentially enhance our lives in many ways. Yang is actually doing it. Having great ideas is easy, we all have them daily, but not many people actually focus in one great idea, dig in, apply themselves, and actually make it real. Those who do usually end up with higher self-esteem than the rest of those who dreamed but never actually did anything about their dream because they gave up too easily or were to unwilling to follow through.

There is a tendency I have noticed in some people to claim that they are not creative in any way and I have found that it is absolute nonsense. Every day, we are creating our lives, we choose our clothes, we choose our foods, we problem solve at work. All of these activities is a creative process. Every moment we are making decisions, do we go with that or this, do I say that, or this. Therefore, creativity is a fundamental part of being human and a direct expression of the yin and yang that flows through us.

The Yin and Yang of Addiction

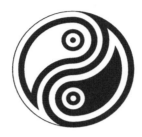

Yang = desire, craving, aversion, compulsive, movement, self-absorbed, obsessive
Yin = content, relaxed, stillness, flexible, not bothered by

Addiction is primarily a yang energetic expression that manifests as a compulsiveness. Addiction can refer to any wanting, needing, craving, or seeking of anything, which may include food, shopping, stimulation, adrenaline, drugs, alcohol, sex, relationships, attention, and so on. Addictions refer to yang energy whereas yin is experienced as the opposite, where the person is not bothered either way because they find contentedness in most, if not all situations. If a yin person gets the object of their desire, good, if they don't get it, that's good, too. Therefore, all addictions are expressions of an extreme form of yang energy and if we continue to feed it and follow it, it often leads to more of the same.

One approach to coming out of the pattern of excessive yang energy addiction is to start bringing in yin energy activities. In this approach, we are not interested, especially during the initial stages, to stop the addictive behavior itself, or go 'cold turkey, as this can lead to explosive consequences. Instead, the suggested approach here is to bring more yin activities into one's life, which starts to balance out the persons energy in a way that the cravings and excessive starts to settle of its own accord. Over time and repeated application of yin energy, the addiction can often dissolve and resolve of its own accord with little resistance or sense of loss. Yin energy practices include relaxation, gentle exercises, conscious breathing, meditation, yin foods, and the capacity to be adaptable and flexible and 'let go' in the face of change.

There is also an important distinction to be made here between wanting, desiring, and craving. It is natural to want or desire something, like to eat when one is hungry or to desire better health or better quality relationships. It's when desire goes to the extreme that turns it into craving, which causes us trouble and destabilizes the mind. Therefore, be careful and aware enough so that you don't let your desires and wants turn into craving and it will save you a lot of stress.

The Yin and Yang of Relationships

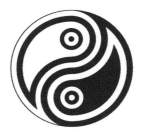

"Balanced relationships are always based on freedom, not obligation." ~ Michael Thomas Sunnarborg

Yang = dynamism, movement, giving, passionate, excitement, expression, talking, superficial
Yin = patience, quietude, relaxation, receiving, contentment, listening, sincere, genuine

Exploring the dynamism of human romantic relationships provides us with a perfect example of yin and yang expressions. Typically, a male has within him a predominant yang source of energy and the female has a more yin source of energy to draw from. This expression of both yin and yang provide the perfect conditions for relationships to flourish, nurture, and develop. It is nature's way to have one person to hold and uphold a predominant yang energy and the other to uphold a more yin energy. This can be seen throughout the animal world, as well as the human world, in the forms of both heterosexual and homosexual relationships.

For a relationship to flourish, a complementary amount of yang or yin energy is required to match the other person's yin or yang energy. For example, if a man upholds 80% yang energy and 20% yin, he would naturally be seeking out a female who expressed 80% yin energy and 20% yang. This is not always the case, however, because some of us, at various stages of our lives, seek out various expressions of yin and yang types of people and this is also a natural process of rebalancing our own energies as a way to rediscover our true state within yin and yang. For example, if we were in a previous relationship with a person who expressed a great amount of yang energy and that relationship finished, then there would probably be a natural tendency to experience and seek out another partner who had more yin as a way to rebalance our system.

There are two types of relationships, one is healthy and supportive whereas the other is harmful and destructive. The former type of relationship is focused on an exchange and sharing of energies to help and support each other toward a higher level of awareness. In this kind of relationship, they often consciously exchange roles, shifting their energy to adjust to the other person. For example, if one person in the relationship has had a difficult day, then the other person shifts their energy and attention to be more accommodating to the other. There is a kind of mutual respect that comes into play that acknowledges the other person's energy and how they are expressing their energies in their daily life.

The other more harmful type of relationship is based in the giving and taking of energy from each other. Usually, one person in the relationship is a taker and the other person is a giver of their energy. The taker cares little for the general well-being of the other person and is only involved in the relationship to serve out their own needs and desires. Takers tend to be predatory in their behaviors, because of the lack of their own self-worth and their inability to generate their own balance and source of energy they seek to steal it from other weakened and vulnerable people. The giver in the relationship has such low self-esteem, for a variety of reasons, from trauma through to poor parental role models, they freely give up their low reserves of energy to feel needed or wanted by the other person. Yet, they know in their hearts that the relationship is not good for them. Relationships that are established and based on this taking and giving of energy from each other is destined for destructive outcomes and should be avoided when possible. In such circumstances, it is better to walk alone than to walk alongside another who seeks to only steal your energy. Having the courage to walk alone can be difficult for people in any circumstance and, therefore, it is advisable for these people to move their focus away from "romantic relationships" and focus on improving their own health and personal energy instead. This helps to bring their internal energy to a more balanced state so that in the future, further relationships will not be based on the giving and taking. When one's energy is internally strengthened and cultivated to the point where you can be self-sustaining and self-dependent, relationships will naturally become more balanced, healthy, and supportive. Until then, it is better to avoid romantic relationships for at least 6 months to a year.

Friendship based relationships tend to take on a different quality of yin and yang, where the friend brings out more of the same in us. For example, if I am a male, running predominantly as a yang energy, there is a tendency to seek out other male friends who also express male dominant characteristics. This generates the sense of being accepted as who you are and it also encourages us to express our natural tendencies. Of course, this is not always the case as we may have one or two close friends who actually show us the other side of yin or yang energy and these friends tend to provide us with a sense of fresh air from the usual circle of friends who all feed on the same energy. Females tend to work much in the same way, and seek out friends who express the same amount of yin dominate energy as themselves. And again, just like males, they may have a good one or two close friends who express the other end of yin or yang, which provide them some insight and freshness into their usual yin dominant friends. In all cases, therefore, it is advisable and natural for us to seek out friends who bring out our true natural expressions of yin or yang energy, yet it is also helpful to be open to those friends who express something very different because it is those friends who help us to stay balanced and provide us insight into the other world, which can be very helpful in providing advice for more romantic focused relationships.

Obvious signs of a yang dominated person is one who:
- Moves fast
- Can be a bit rough around the edges
- Tends to get hot easily
- Wants things to happen quickly and can easily become impatient and frustrated
- Loves to move, dance, exercise
- Loves to talk
- Eats fast
- Seeks out thrills and flashy entertainment
- Extroverted tendencies
- Masculine body shape
- Strong body and frame
- Strong sexual drive

Obvious signs of a yin dominated person is one who:
- Moves slowly
- Likes smooth and soft things
- Warm or cool to the touch
- Is patient
- Is a good listener
- Intuitive, creative

- Enjoys quiet time
- Introverted tendencies
- Often intellectual
- Feminine body shape

The Yin and Yang of Spirituality

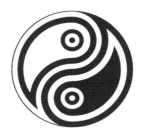

Yang = seeking, learning, studying, trying to "get it", effort, passion, fire, ritual, experimenting with techniques, repetitious practicing, practicing with goals, the world of forms, doctrine, external source

Yin = non-seeking, knowingness, stillness, meditative, contemplative, teaching through presence, effortlessness, embodied, practicing with no goal, the world of non-form, internal realization, internal source

Spirituality is a major component of the human being and, therefore, it is worth exploring in the context of yin and yang. Yang in regard to spirituality refers to actively seeking out understanding and to be one who is considered a seeker. Yin fully embodies knowingness without the effort and is experienced when the seeking is surrendered.

The yang of spirituality can easily be linked to various religious practices, rituals, and techniques. The tendency of the seeker is to be heavily focused on these techniques and rituals, which is often a reflection that the seeker is seeking spiritual truth, information, and salvation via outside sources. Religions have a tendency to be heavily depended on stories and dramatizations from a past time as well as using great promises for future time. Spirituality, in contrast, is more so focused on the presence truth of now. Spiritual truth, therefore, arises from within and is not interested in the past or the future.

Initially for the spiritual aspirate, it is natural to go through the yang stages of spirituality endeavor first. As we experience willingness, curiosity, and the searching for truth and deeper meanings in our lives, we reorient our lives so as to pursue a greater spiritual understanding that expresses as yang energy. The aspirant may join a local spiritual group, learn new techniques, and study scriptures as a way to gain greater spiritual understanding and this is normal.

There are many traps and obstacles on the spiritual path, mainly put up by the ego-mind and the spiritual ego, which serve to throw us off course or fill us with a false understanding. Why does our own ego try to throw us off the scent? Because the ego-mind loses its power over us the more we come to understand our true nature and our true spirituality. Instead of an ego-mind dominating our perceptions of the world, a deeper, inner spiritual power starts to awaken within and over time, it develops to such a state that it overpowers our ego-mind and a great knowingness takes it place, which is the yin essence. For a human being who has attained such a state of knowingness, they may still carry out various spiritual practices in their daily life, yet their orientation has changed and they do it not as a way to seek or attain anything, but as a way to honor and show gratitude for what is known. Therefore, the yang of spirituality is the orientation of seeking something whereas the yin of spirituality is giving thanks for what already is.

Bringing More Yin In

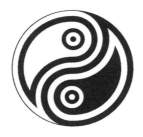

The overarching theme of yin promoting activities and attitudes tends to be that which promotes slowing down, the reduction of stimulation, quiet, stillness, and the activation of the parasympathetic nervous system. This chapter is dedicated to practical methods and techniques to promote more yin in our lives, especially suited and recommended to those who show signs of being yang dominant.

Initially, when installing new habits and activities into our lives, it is better to do it gradually and progressively rather than all at once. Humans tend to resist dramatic and sudden change and it has been found that humans tend to do things more effectively and sustainably when practices and habit are introduced slowly. Introducing one or two new practices or habits every 20 – 30 days has been shown to increase the chance that it will "stick" and so this provides us with a suitable guideline.

- Avoid taking on any more commitments or projects and even seek to remove one or two so to encourage more space in your life. Allows more free time to open up.

- Emotional Freedom Technique (EFT) tapping on acupressure points at least once a day to reduce the intensity of stress and tensions in the body.

- Slowly reduce excessive consumption of highly acidic foods.

- Avoid enforcing your personal will into a situation. This often causes unnecessary conflict and shows lack of trust in the universal will. It is better to stay calm and relaxed in the current moment and let the external factors organize themselves. The more we learn to let go of that type of enforcing, the more things tend to turn out for the better, of all those involved.

-Watch less TV, less movies, and reduce amount of time spent on computers and digital devices. Instead, read books, listen to more relaxing music, go for a walk, spend more time with people who support yin energy, and spend more time in nature.

- Receive a massage or acupuncture treatment at least once a month.

- Introduce slow form exercises like tai chi or gentle yoga.

On the following pages are a list of yoga postures that promote yin.

Butterfly Pose

1. Bring the soles of your feet together. Allow some space between the heels of your feet and your groin—no need to jam yourself up.

2. Grab your feet, or interlace your fingers around your toes (it doesn't really matter which); inhale to lengthen through your spine, exhale to draw yourself gently forward and down.

3. Take your time to soften into the pose. Connective tissue in the body takes at least thirty seconds to respond, so just go easy into it.

4. After thirty seconds to one minute, allow your back to curl and your head to soften toward the floor. Let gravity do the work! Relax your shoulders, arms, legs, and head, and sink toward the floor. Closing the eyes can be very powerful here. Stay for at least three minutes if comfortable.

5. For extra comfort and support, use a yoga bolster to rest your head on. When the body feels the support, it will naturally begin to release and relax. Keep your breath smooth and gentle. Stay for at least three minutes if comfortable; if not comfortable, then come up whenever you're ready.

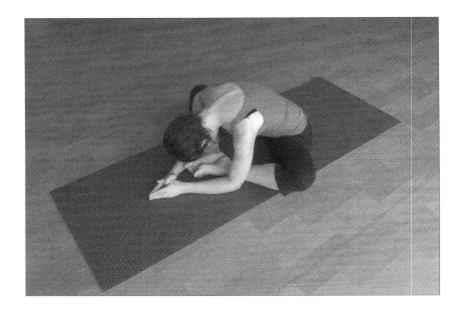

Forward Bend

1. Sit with your legs straight out in front of you.

2. Place the bolster (or a few pillows) on your thighs. Be sure not to cramp your belly area; give it some space.

3. When you're ready, simply inhale, draw the arms above the head, and get some length on the spine. Then, as you exhale, draw your chest forward and down over the legs. You don't have to be able to grab your feet—that's not important. Your hands go anywhere that is comfortable; on the floor, on your legs, or on your feet is fine.

4. Take your time and be patient. It takes a while for some tissues in the body to respond, so just keep breathing and keep softening into it. We want to reach a point where gravity is doing most of

the work for you; you just have to soften your body and allow it to move further down toward the floor. Relax your shoulders and arms, no need to hold on here…

5. Allow the back to curl, and relax your head to rest the forehead onto the bolster or pillows. Close the eyes, soften the body, and breathe. Hold for at least three minutes if comfortable. Feel free to come out if you feel like you've had enough. (Try not to come out until you have found at least one moment of peace within the pose.)

Variations:

1. If you are having difficulty getting your chest and torso forward, then try sitting up on some blankets or some cushions so your hips are off the floor. This helps the upper body to be able to come forward over the legs. Experiment with the height of the hips if you need to. With this one, you are looking to find a place where gravity takes over and draws your torso down toward the legs.

2. If you have trouble getting your head to sit on the bolster or the pillows, you may need to increase the amount of pillows and cushions so that your head can find a place to rest on them. If that is too distracting, or you don't have enough pillows to make it work, try not using any pillows or supports and letting your head hang in space toward the floor. Relax your neck and let gravity draw your head down. Breathe. Soften.

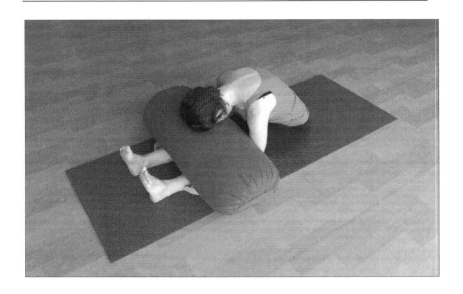

Reclining Bridge

This is one of my favorites. This is an amazing pose to release the lower back, and it sends blood and nutrients to the lungs, heart, and brain.

To set yourself up for this pose, you will need a bolster or some big blocky cushions. Pillows are unlikely to be enough here. Bring the bolster or blocky cushions lengthwise down the mat, so that your hips and legs can be supported and off the floor, like in the picture above.

1. To get into position, line up the bolster, and maybe add an extra pillow, cushion, or bolster if you have long legs, like me.

2. Sit up and straddle the bolster, with legs on either side. Then start to lie back. Make sure the bolster sits nicely into the lower back, supporting the sacrum. Don't let it come up so it is touching your ribs. You want it lower than that, so it sits nicely in

the lower back curve. Your shoulders should easily rest on the floor or mat. You can use a folded blanket under the head if you need the extra support.

3. Bring the legs up onto the bolster. You will need to bring the legs comfortably together, and let the feet splay out to the sides.

4. Relax the arms down the side of the body and soften the back of the neck.

5. Stay for at least 3 – 5 minutes. Take your time. Close your eyes. Breathe gently.

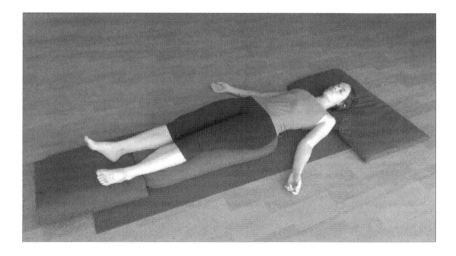

Variation:

1. Sometimes the legs won't stay up on the bolster, as they can slip off the sides. If you have this issue, then, when you are straddling the bolster and ready to lie back, try strapping your legs together around the calf muscles with a yoga strap or a belt. Keep your

knees bent so you can recline more easily. When your back is settled on the floor, extend the legs out on top of the bolster. Then recline down toward the mat, and when your back is settled, bring the legs up to rest on the bolster. Let the feet splay out to the sides. The strap should hold the legs together so you can really let go of the legs.

Legs Up the Wall

This is a great pose to start off with, especially if you have been on your feet all day. It drains the feet and flushes the organs with blood and nutrients. This is a safe variation for all.

1. Getting into this position can be a bit awkward. If you have a bolster available, keep it close and within arm's reach. However, if you don't have a bolster, it doesn't matter because keeping your hips on the mat is good, too. To start, the key is to sit up alongside a wall, getting as close as you can to the wall with one hip.

2. Then, roll yourself down onto your back and shoot your legs up the wall. Ideally, the buttocks are quite close to the wall, though people who have tight hamstrings will need to come away from the wall so they can get their legs up. In this case, the knees will probably be bent, but that's okay. If your hamstrings are okay, wiggle yourself closer to the wall so your buttocks touch the wall.

3. If you want to add the bolster for extra support, then grab the bolster and bring it close to your hips. Place your feet onto the wall and push the feet into the wall so you can raise your buttocks and hips off the floor slightly. Then quickly slide the bolster under where your hips would be if they were on the floor. Then lower your hips down onto the bolster. Once you find a

comfortable position, let your arms fall away to the side, close your eyes, and just relax with a gentle breath. You can stay here for 3 – 15 minutes.

4. To come out, bend the knees, then roll to your right side. Wait here for a minute or two so the legs can get some blood back into them before moving or standing. Take your time... if the phone rings or something like this, let it go... do not rush out of this one.

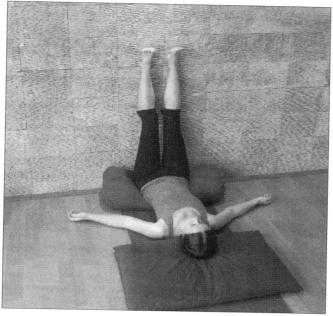

Variations:

1. If the hamstrings are tight, just wiggle yourself away from the wall until you find a comfortable position where your legs can rest against the wall. Your knees will probably be bent, but that's okay.

2. <u>Sometimes, the legs want to fall away to the sides,</u> and it's hard to relax them because you have to hold them up there. If this happens, you can strap your legs together with a yoga strap, a belt, or anything really. Strap them together around the calf muscle area. To do this, when you get onto your back, bend your knees into your chest, and then strap the legs together. When done, extend them up the wall and wiggle yourself into a comfortable position.

3. <u>Simply bring the soles of the feet together and let the knees fall out to the side.</u>

Shavasana (corpse pose)

This is the pose you always need to finish any sequence with. The body needs a moment to settle and reorganize itself. It is very powerful and should not be skipped over. Even just one minute can bring much benefit. There are many variations to this pose, but one thing remains consistent – the total relaxation of the body in the supine position.

1. Lie straight out on the floor with your legs extended.

2. Place legs slightly apart, with feet splaying out to the sides.

3. Your arms should lie just away from the body, with palms facing up or down. Or, you can place your palms onto your chest or belly, whichever feels right for you.

4. Close your eyes. Relax the eyes into the sockets.

5. Have a quick scan through your body, moving your awareness through your feet, legs, hips, back, belly, chest, arms, shoulders, neck, and head. Check to make sure that you're not holding on to any tension in the body.

6. Stay for 1 – 5 minutes. Try not to move your body; just remain still. Relinquish thoughts as they arise; don't give them any importance, just let them go for now.

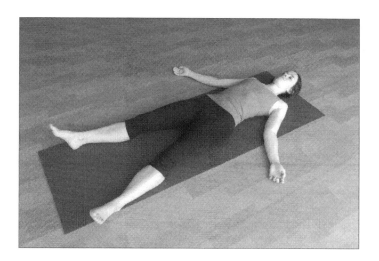

Variations:

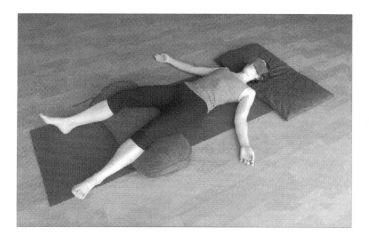

1. You might like to try bringing a bolster or pillow supports under the knees. This helps soften the lower back toward the floor. Therefore, this is <u>recommended if you have lower back pain</u> or problems. Also, if you have an eye pillow, now is a good time to use it. Something placed under the back of head to raise the head slightly off the floor can help relax the muscles in the neck. However, avoid big fluffy pillows because they can raise the head too high and create strain in the neck.

2. Follow steps 3 – 6.

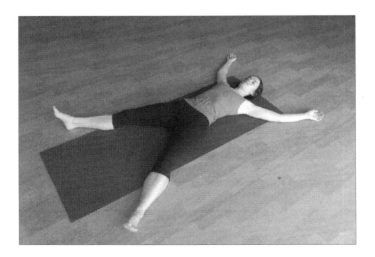

1. Find a comfortable position by bringing the arms out diagonally above the head and widen the legs slightly.

2. Close your eyes and let your body completely rest for at least 1-5 minutes.

Bringing More Yang In

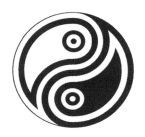

Yang activities and practices tend to steer us toward those things that promote the more invigorating, stimulating, and fiery qualities in us. It is necessary to have a little yang here and there in our lifestyles but it can easily become harmful if we get hooked on it and let it blow out to the extreme. Therefore, always trod cautiously with yang, as yang is quick to react and respond whereas yin is slower to respond.

Because of its fast and explosive nature, yang imbalances are lot quicker to respond and treat. It is much easier to bring up the yang in someone to override their predominantly yin characteristics than it is to put out the yang and build the yin quality.

Regardless, yang is an essential part of our makeup and is required to bring success in this material world for money is naturally drawn to those who have the energy of willingness that comes from a yang type energy. To put it simply, those who tend to have success with the material world, which includes wealth, are willing to do what is necessary to become more attractive in their careers and relationships. Willingness, therefore, requires yang energy, knowledge, focus, persistence, and discipline.

Ways to generate more yang:

- Write up a list of goals and aspirations. Include: what do you want to learn, what skills do you want to have, where do you want to visit, who do you want to meet? Also, what are your short term goals (1-3 years) and divide it into 3 sections. Your economic goals, your stuff and things goals, and your personal development goals. Do the same for your long term goals 5-10 years. This gives us the energy of excitement and motivation and sets us on a trajectory into the future. Take your time to do this and ponder over it carefully. Every month, revisit the document and tick off those ones you have achieved.

- Become more active in your learning. It is not necessary to always think of learning and study as in terms of university or college. These days it is very easy and possible to self study and become very intelligent and "clued in" from this process. In fact, I personally have found self-directed study to be more valuable than university directed study.

- Get focused.

- Introduce more stimulating and dynamic forms of movement and exercise, it could be dancing, running, and/or yang forms of yoga.

- Surround yourself with motivational and successful people

- Eat less dairy and heavy greasy foods, while eating more spicy, well cooked foods.

The following pages have a list of some yoga poses that stimulate yang energy:

Sun Salutations

Repeat this sequence at least x3 most days. Morning time is generally the best time to practice.

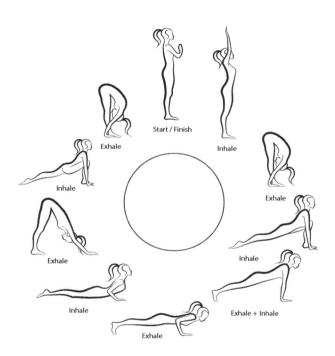

Down Facing Dog – Adho Mukha Svanasana

1. Come onto all fours with hands underneath the shoulders and knees under the hips. Spread your fingers wide.

2. Tuck the toes under, start to extend the arms and start bringing the knees off the floor
3. Come to extend the arms and start to work the legs straight. Try to bring the weight back into your legs and not so much into your arms.
4. Look to the floor just under your belly button.

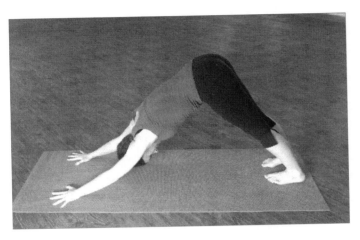

Low Lunge – Anjaneyasana

1. Ideally, you will start in a standing-forward, bent position (Uttanasana) at the front of the mat. Then simply step your left leg to the back of the mat and bring your back knee to the floor; the top of your back foot should be flat on the floor.
2. Make sure your front ankle is either just in front of or directly underneath your front knee.
3. Open your heart up and bring your arms out to the side, and then bring them up above your head. In this picture, the hands are shoulder width apart—this makes it easier to relax the shoulders down away from the ears. You can bring your hands together too, if that feels more natural.
4. Allow your lower back to lengthen and gently work your hips forward and down toward the floor, opening the front of your left hip.

5. After a few breaths, bring your torso and your arms down toward the floor, tuck your back toe under and step to the front of the mat, returning to your forward bend at the front of the mat.

6. Repeat on the other side.

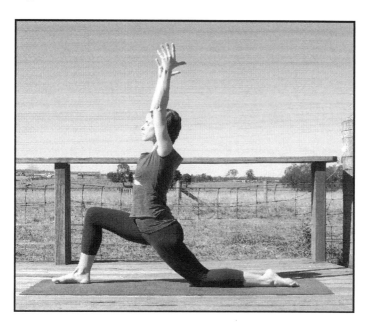

Locust - Salabhasana

1. Lie on your belly in the middle of your mat.

2. Bring the arms down the side of the body, palms facing up. Feet hip width apart. Looking forward, resting the head on the chin.

3. On an inhale, start to raise the upper body, the arms, and hands off the floor. Try to get the arms parallel with the floor.

4. Then start to raise the legs off the floor. Try to keep your legs straight.

5. Look diagonally down toward the floor to keep the neck in line with the spine.

6. Now gently squeeze the hands toward each other so you activate the muscles around the shoulder blades.

8. Keep the breath moving. Hold for 3-4 breaths and then slowly release and relax back onto your mat.

9. Have a little rest for a few moments and do it at least one more time.

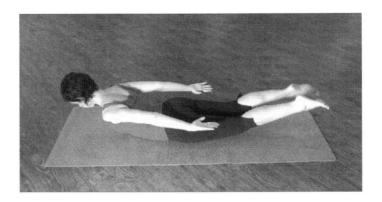

Extended Side Angle Pose - Utthita Parsva Konasana

1. Extend the legs wide apart and bring your right toe to face down the mat and the back toes to turn out to the side at around 45 degrees.

2. Bring your hands to your hips to start with and start to bend into the front right knee. Make sure your knee is either above your ankle or just behind it, don't let it pass over the ankle as this puts too much stress on the knee joint.

3. Bring your arms up to shoulder height, shoulders relaxed, and palms facing down.

4. Now start to reach forward with your right arm, bring your torso forward also, and then place the right elbow onto the knee.

Bring the left arms past your ear, palm facing down. Look out to the side or up under the arm.

5. Keep your legs strong, draw the belly in, try and relax the upper body.

6. Come out by drawing the arms and torso back to center, and releasing the legs.

7. Repeat on other side

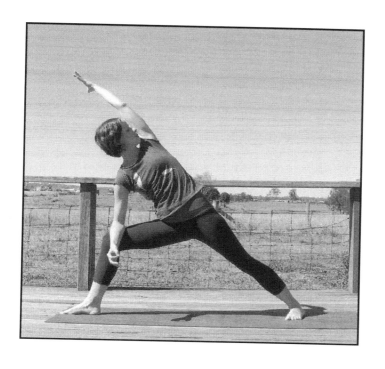

Horse Stance – Arms pushing Qi out to the side

1. Bring your legs comfortable apart, feet at 45 degrees and start to sink into the knees a little. Get the sense that the knees are working outwards and work big toes into the floor.

2. Allow the tailbone to gently move toward the floor, yet a low a gentle lower back curve. Basically, no jamming into the lower back. Draw the anus in slightly and get a sense that the lower belly is drawn in slightly – you want to feel strong in your lower body, like a tree.

3. The arms, the branches, gently push out to the sides, shoulders and elbows soft so the energy can flow easily.

4. Eyes forward, relaxed face. Close down the eyes and breathe and hold for a few minutes.

5. Keep lower body strong and upper body light – you will feel the Qi intensify after a minute or two.

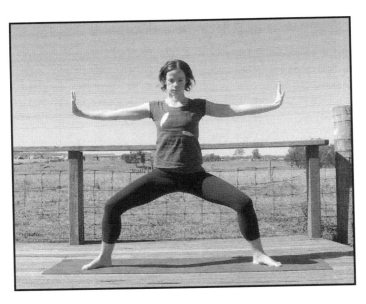

Beyond Yin and Yang

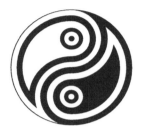

"Out beyond ideas of wrong doing and right doing, there is a field; I will meet you there." ~ Rumi

Exploring yin and yang is useful to help us navigate the universal laws of these two opposing forces but we all will eventually come to a point where we ask: Can we go beyond the forces of yin and yang?

The answer, in simple terms, is yes. The transcendence of the force of yin and yang takes place only on the spiritual level. When a person has passed through the yang to unveil the yin essence of spirituality, they transcend yin and yang. As mentioned briefly in the introduction of this book, the most common path tends to be via the maturation and development of the mind until one reaches a point where they have an opportunity to leap beyond it. Leaping beyond the mind takes us to the space of the spiritual essence that encompasses all the aspects of the mind. Although some of us will have the opportunity to get established in living from the spirit realm, because the density of the physical body and the subtle nature of mind energy, these aspects of the human being are still under the influence of yin and yang. Yet, when the person's spirit is firmly established in the space beyond yin and yang, the forces of yin still play out on the body and mind, yet it does not trouble or disturb them. It's as if they become just a witness to these movements as opposed to being moved by them directly. In fact, our spiritual nature is already in a perpetual space beyond yin and yang forces, although, most humans are not aware of this place and hence, we are primarily thrown around and governed via the yin and yang influencing upon our bodies and minds.

The spiritual aspirant does not seek to run away from the influencing forces of yin and yang, but instead, seeks to understand them so thoroughly that that it produces an enhanced capacity to move beyond them.

Conclusion

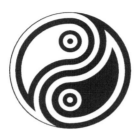

" When I let go of what I am, I become what I might be."
~ Lao Tzu

Yin and yang provide us with one of the simplest and most practical applications to study and understand the forces of nature. Through the study and ongoing alignment with the natures if yin and yang, life dissolves of its struggles and a smoother and more fluid path appears. Thus, the purpose of this book, and this work, is to help all those who are interested, curious, and willing, to enliven and illuminate their path with greater understanding and with greater ease.

The philosophy of yin and yang is one of the oldest contributions to humanity, yet its deeper understandings have been distorted and lost in time. And so the modern man seems to be rushing here and there, without much guidance or direction, becoming lost in the maze of his own mind. With the application of yin and yang into our daily life, we can more readily tap into an energy source much greater than our own personal will that can not only serve as a guide but also dissolve a great deal of struggle and avoid the loss of energy.

From the outlined subjects in this book, I sincerely hope that you now have a more thorough understanding as to how to work with and align with yin and yang. An important factor to always remember is that yin and yang forces are not personal. They do not care about our opinions, our beliefs, or religious tendencies, because yin and yang operate as they do, regardless. Therefore, it is wise to continue to explore and experiment with similar universal truths and rely less upon opinions or belief systems to guide your focus and energy.

Yin and yang are here to help you in enhancing all aspects of your life, if you are open and willing to align with them. When we are able to catch these cosmic yin and yang waves as they move through us and our environment, immense power is available that can uplift and support us, therefore making anything possible. It is exciting to know that we all have this powerful energy available to us. The only requirement is to learn to groove, dance, and flow with it. After reading the pages of this book, this will be much clearer and easier for you.

May your journey be fruitful and uplifted via the life giving forces of yin and yang.

~ May all beings be happy ~

Other Books By This Author

www.michaelhetherington.com.au

The Complete Book of Oriental Yoga

Meditation Made Simple

How to Do Restorative Yoga

Chakra Balancing Made Simple and Easy

The Little Book of Yin

How to Learn Acupuncture

Printed in Great Britain
by Amazon

61369961R00066